Mediterranean Diet Cookbook For Beginners

1500 Days of Affordable and Mouthwatering Recipes to Change Your Eating Lifestyle Forever. Bonus: 30-Day Flexible Meal Plan On a Budget

Gloria Reiber

TABLE OF CONTENTS

Introduction

The Mediterranean diet is, at its heart, a healthy way of eating that is rich in vegetables and fruit, fish and seafood, whole grains and legumes. The Mediterranean diet has been linked to a reduced risk of cancer, diabetes, heart disease and Alzheimer's. A study published in the American Journal of Preventive Medicine found that people who followed the Mediterranean diet have nearly 20% less chance of dying from cardiovascular disease compared to those following other diets. People who eat at least five servings of fruits or vegetables daily are recommended for the best protection against chronic diseases such as dementia or cancer.

A Mediterranean diet rich in fruit and vegetables, seafood, meat and dairy products has been proven to benefit cholesterol levels, as well as reduce the risk of many serious diseases. A recent study done in 2004 in Greece where researchers observed over 26,000 people concluded that those who followed the "Mediterranean lifestyle" for less than five years had a 14% lower mortality rate (death) compared to those who lived healthier but did not follow the Mediterranean lifestyle.

The benefits of a Mediterranean diet are well documented by large-scale studies in population groups. However, until now it has not been possible to link specific aspects of the Mediterranean diet with specific health effects. The new study by the Helmholz association in Germany sought to test whether certain aspects of the Mediterranean diet have a direct role in protecting from cardiovascular disease or Alzheimer's disease.

An increasing number of epidemiological studies have proven that people who are obese (having a BMI above 30) or those with a high waist circumference have an increased risk for heart disease, high cholesterol and diabetes. Being overweight is also associated with an increased risk of developing dementia and other incurable diseases like cancer.

The new study evaluated data from the German health survey (DKfZ), which is a large representative study that has collected data from over 10,000 people in Germany. The participants had all filled out a detailed questionnaire regarding their lifestyles and diet.

The "Mediterranean lifestyle" was defined as a diet rich in fruits, vegetables and fish and low in animal protein. They were further subdivided into three groups based on their degree of adherence to these dietary guidelines:

1. Mediterranean diet with less than 1 serving per day of white bread, pasta or rice (less than 25% of energy intake)

2. Mediterranean diet with 1–3 servings per day of white bread, pasta or rice (25–49%)

3. Mediterranean diet with 4 to 6 servings per day of white bread, pasta or rice (50–75%)

The researchers found that people following the Mediterranean diet on average get all their dietary recommendations in terms of amounts, but more fruits and vegetables are recommended for the more strict adherence. The findings from a previous study from 2006 by the same Helmholz association have been confirmed in this new study: people who follow a Mediterranean diet have nearly 20% less chance of dying from cardiovascular disease compared to those following other diets.

In scientific studies, death is measured as all deaths which were not caused by diabetes, cancer or stroke.

The data showed that the women who followed a Mediterranean diet had a lower risk of death from any cause, compared to those who follow other diets. Also, the researchers found that people following the Mediterranean diet but with no high adherence to the other dietary recommendations had a significantly reduced risk of death from any cause compared to those following other diets.

The study has not yet been published and has not been peer reviewed by other scientists. However, the findings are in line with previous studies suggesting that a Mediterranean diet may be associated with healthy aging and reduced mortality in people over 65 years old.

Brief history

The Mediterranean diet is one of the best diets out there. The Mediterranean-style diet is often considered one of the healthiest, yet most delicious ways to eat. Greek salads, Italian pasta dishes and fresh seafood are just some of the many staples on a Mediterranean menu.

The Mediterranean diet is a diet that can easily be followed by anyone, yet it is most popular in countries bordering the Mediterranean Sea. The Mediterranean diet focuses on whole foods, including grains, fruits and vegetables. It also focuses on healthy fats and proteins. Dairy, legumes and sweets are eaten in moderation. Grains are mostly whole grains such as breads, couscous and pasta. Fruits are eaten fresh or dried while vegetables are eaten in abundance. Olive oil is the main source of fat with other fats coming mainly from fish and nuts. Meats include poultry, eggs, lean beef and low-fat dairy products with very little red meat eaten in most regions. Meats are eaten in small amounts over the course of a week. A typical Mediterranean diet meal consists of at least 5 ounces of seafood, plenty of fresh fruits, vegetables and whole grains.

The original version of the Mediterranean diet was developed by a Greek physician named Adonis in the late 1800s. The original Mediterranean Diet consisted primarily of fats from olive oil, fish and nuts with some fruits and whole grains. Later modifications to the Mediterranean diet include a focus on plant-based foods and greater inclusion of dairy products such as yogurt and cheese. Many sections of the Mediterranean diet retain high levels of fat, yet lower levels are present in most modern versions. However, the traditional version was closer to the current version.

The Mediterranean diet has been shown to be beneficial in many ways. In addition to **Nutrition**al benefits, a Mediterranean-style diet also leads to weight loss and has anti-inflammatory properties. This can be attributed to the high fiber content in foods such as vegetables and whole grains as well as healthy fats. It is important that people eat vegetables in order to get all of the nutrients they need and eliminate their risk of cancer and heart disease.

Many studies show that individuals who eat a Mediterranean-style diet have lower amounts of inflammation throughout their bodies than those who do not. A Mediterranean-style diet is also linked to better immunity and cardiovascular health.

Besides the benefits of the Mediterranean diet, it is also important that people receive adequate amounts of fiber in their diets. Fiber helps with weight loss and can help with the prevention of certain diseases such as cancer, diabetes and heart disease. Consuming foods such as vegetables, fruits, whole grains and legumes can help someone get enough fiber in their diets. By eating more vegetables and fruits, a person can get enough fiber into their diets without having to add extra sugar or high fat foods because they will not be a large source of calories for the body.

The Benefits of the Mediterranean Diet

Improves Heart Health

The study shows that a Mediterranean diet rich in ALA (alpha-linolenic acid) found in olive oil can decrease the risk of cardiac death in a person by nearly 30. Further research shows that when comparing the blood pressure between people who consumed sunflower oil versus those consuming extra virgin oil, the olive oil consumers were able to decrease their blood pressure by more significant amounts.

Weight Loss

The types of food that the Mediterranean diet encourages, such as whole grains, beans, and legumes, consist of high amounts of fiber, which help to slow digestion and prevent frequent spikes in blood sugar levels. This means you feel full for a longer period without needing a snack.

Mediterranean diet is less caloric than the fatty diet of many western countries, and it makes large use of aromatic herbs that allow you to flavor the dishes, which has little or no amounts of fatty and high-calorie condiments.

Can Help to Fight Cancer

A study at the Mayo Clinic found that 800 people with advanced colon polyps ate red meat more frequently, and their diet did not correspond to foods on the Mediterranean diet. The World Cancer Research Fund reports that eating at least 90 grams of whole grains a day can lessen your risk of colon cancer by almost 20%. This is because the fiber in whole grains prevents any mutations from developing in your digestive tract and keeps your bowel movement in check.

Lowers Risk of Cardiovascular Disease

The Mediterranean diet has been acknowledged to be most helpful in reducing high triglyceride levels. Triglycerides are fatty molecules that travel throughout the bloodstream and build up plaque in our arteries. A higher triglyceride count or its accumulation in the bloodstream and vessels can lead to greater chance of stroke or heart attack and cholesterol. Even though the Mediterranean diet consists of fatty items like olive oil and salmon, they are good fats that are loaded with beneficial monounsaturated and polyunsaturated fats.

Protects Cognitive Health

Following the Mediterranean diet could be key in protecting yourself from future neurodegenerative diseases like Parkinson's, dementia, or Alzheimer's. The healthy fats that the Mediterranean diet is full of are known to fight age-related cognitive decline, along with the anti-inflammatory protection that fresh fruits and vegetables provide.

It can improve your memory, mental acuity, and attention span as it protects your nerve cells from deteriorating with age.

Protection Against Type-2 Diabetes

The Mediterranean diet encourages meals seasoned with healthy spices and also encourages you to fill your dessert with fruit instead of baked foods that contain sugar. It is also significant that in many studies, participants on the Mediterranean diet tended to lose, on average more weight than participants on other low carb or low-fat diets. Due to this weight loss, you can reduce your risk of diabetes, and maybe even delay needing any further medication.

Increase Sight

Since the Mediterranean diet is full of fruits, vegetables, and regular servings of fish, it has great amounts of vitamins that protect your sight. Fish is also high in omega-three fatty acids, which is critical to sight health. Just having one serving of fish in a week can lower the risk of developing eye damage, which occurs commonly in people over the age of 50. With the Mediterranean diet, you are incorporating fish in your diet more than two times a week! The seeds and nuts you are eating as snacks also contain fatty acids that protect the retinas from cellular damage, which occurs with age.

Your Kidney Function Improves

A 2014 study in the Clinical Journal of American Society of Nephrology found that following the Mediterranean diet may decrease the chances of having chronic kidney disease by almost 50%. This could be attributed to clean and healthy food choices that the Mediterranean diet requires, with less processed food and red meat. Fish, nuts, fresh fruits, and vegetables are known to lower inflammation in the body, which causes kidney disease.

Keeps Your Skin Healthy

By following the Mediterranean diet, you will cut out extra sugar and instead rely on healthy fruits with natural sugars. A study even found that people with higher blood sugar levels were considered "older-looking" based on the appearance of their skin compared to people with low blood sugar levels. Eating a balanced diet full of healthy vitamins and minerals keeps your skin healthy, and that's precisely what the Mediterranean diet provides!

What To Eat: The Mediterranean Diet Food List

The Mediterranean diet is a very beneficial diet. That said, it is very hard for you to experience any of the benefits that you have just learned without following the diet to the latter. One way of doing that is by eating what the diet allows and avoiding what the diet prohibits you to eat. Let's get started

Foods to eat

The foods you can eat while you are on a Mediterranean diet fall into two categories. There are those foods that you can eat regularly and there are those that you should only eat in moderation. Here is an extensive list of both categories.

Foods to eat regularly

Healthy fats like avocado oil, avocados, olives and extra virgin olive oil

Fruits like peaches, figs, melons, dates, bananas, strawberries, grapes, pears, oranges, and apples. Note that you can eat most fruits while on this diet

Vegetables like cucumbers, Brussels sprouts, artichoke, eggplant, carrots, cauliflower, onions, spinach, kale, broccoli and tomatoes. Those are just popular examples but basically all vegetables are allowed in the Mediterranean diet

Whole grains like pasta, whole wheat, whole grain bread, corn, buckwheat, barley, rye, brown rice and whole oats.

Nuts and seeds like pumpkin seeds, cashews, pistachios, walnuts, almonds and macadamia nuts

Herbs and spices; the best herbs and spices are mostly fresh and dried like mint, rosemary, cinnamon, basil and pepper.

Tubers like sweet potatoes, yams, turnips and potatoes.

Legumes like chickpeas, peanuts, pulses, lentils, peas and beans.

Fish and seafood, which are actually your primary source of protein. Good examples include shellfish like crab, mussels and oysters, shrimp, tuna, haddock and salmon.

Foods You Should Eat In Moderation

You should only eat the below foods less frequently when compared to the foods in the list above.

Red meat like bacon, ground beef and steak

Dairy products low in fat or fat free. Some of the popular examples include cheese, yogurt and low fat milk

Eggs, as they are good sources of proteins and are healthier when poached and boiled

Poultry like duck, turkey and chicken

Note that chicken are healthy when their skin is removed. This is because you reduce the cholesterol in the chicken.

Later on in the book, this list of foods that you are allowed to eat when on a Mediterranean diet will be expanded further where you will know what foods to take on a daily, weekly and monthly basis.

Food to Avoid

The below list contains a couple of foods that you need to avoid when on a Mediterranean diet completely. This is because they are unhealthy and when you eat them, you will be unable to experience the benefits of a Mediterranean diet. These foods include;

Processed meat- you should avoid processed meats like bacon, sausage and hot dogs because they are high in saturated fats, which are unhealthy.

Refined oils - stay away from unhealthy oils like cottonseed oil, vegetable oil and soybean oil.

Saturated or Trans-fats - good example of these fats include butter and margarine.

Highly processed foods – avoid all highly processed foods. By this, I mean all the foods that are packaged. This can be packaged crisp, nuts, wheat etc. Some of these foods are marked and labeled low fat but are actually quite high in sugar.

Refined grains - avoid refined grains like refined pasta, white bread, cereals, bagels etc.

Added sugar- foods, which contain added sugar like sodas, chocolates, candy and ice cream should be completely avoided. If you have a sweet tooth, you can substitute products with added sugar with natural sweeteners.

Now that you know what to eat and what not to eat when on the Mediterranean diet you are now ready to learn how you can adopt the diet. The next chapter will show you how to do that.

Shopping list

Extra-virgin olive oil

The Mediterranean diet as a whole consists of numerous dietary patterns, but olive oil is the foundation of each one. Tocopherols, carotenoids, and polyphenols, which are abundant in extra-virgin olive oil, give it antioxidant and anti-inflammatory qualities. This culinary essential is equally useful for everyday staples like dips, spreads, and salad dressings as it is for cooking. Look for an olive oil in a dark bottle while buying for premium olive oil. The tinting helps preserve the delicate fats from being rancid because light and heat may do this. Once you get your oil home, keep it cool and dark to maintain its quality.

Fresh fruits and veggies

In Mediterranean cuisine, seasonal, locally grown ingredients is emphasized. Frittatas, beans, and lentil soups frequently include dark leafy greens like kale, beet greens, mustard greens, and collard greens. Additionally popular in both cooked and raw dishes are wild greens like dandelion, chicory, and rocket. Artichokes, beets, broccoli, cucumber, eggplant, mushrooms, radishes, and onions are some additional vegetables grown in this area. A staple of Mediterranean cuisine is garlic, which is utilized as a versatile flavoring in everything from sauces and soups to grain meals (and it packs some impressive health benefits).

Apples, apricots, avocados, berries, citrus, dates, figs, grapes, stone fruit, and pomegranates are among the fruits frequently seen in the Mediterranean diet. Lemon juice is frequently squeezed over seafood, vegetables ,soups and beans for a fresh finish.

Fresh herbs and spices

Cooking in the Mediterranean region frequently uses fragrant herbs and spices. In addition to providing antioxidants that are good for your health, these plant-based seasonings eliminate the need for excessive salt. Although the flavors of the Mediterranean vary from place to region, you can bet on parsley, basil, oregano, coriander, and bay leaves to feature frequently. Make homemade pesto with fresh basil or a tangy gremolata with a bunch of parsley.

Fresh and canned seafood

In the Mediterranean diet, fish and shellfish are important sources of protein and good fats. Fresh or canned, omega-3-rich fish including tuna, sardines, and salmon are favorites. Pasta and grain recipes sometimes include mussels, clams, and shrimp. They can also be served plain with lemon, olive oil, and herbs. Most Mediterranean diets recommend eating fish twice a week.

Whole grains

The staple grain of the Mediterranean is wheat. One of Italy's traditional grains, farro is utilized in both hot recipes and cold salads. Bulgur, which is produced from broken wheat berries and used in pilafs and tabbouleh, is another traditional grain. Barley, couscous, and pasta are other common foods across the globe. Look for "whole" or similar terms when purchasing whole grains.

Legumes (dried and canned)

The chickpea, which is made into hummus, falafel, and salads, is one of the most common pulses in Mediterranean cuisine. For flavorful one-pot meals that are rich in protein and fiber, lentils are frequently added to soups and stews. Black-eyed peas, kidney beans, and cannellini beans are frequently added to salads along with a squeeze of fresh lemon and a sprinkle of olive oil.

Nuts and seeds

Due to their trinity of fiber, protein, and fat, nuts and seeds make a filling snack. Tahini, a condiment prepared from powdered sesame seeds, is a staple along the Mediterranean coast. This adaptable condiment, well known for its usage in hummus, also enhances salad dressings.

Olives and capers

Table olives are eaten as a straightforward snack or to go with a platter of crudités. The most widely consumed olives are kalamata olives, which are frequently used to Greek salads, pasta dishes, and tapenades. Olives are a great source of heart-healthy lipids and antioxidant polyphenols. Capers, whether they are dried or brined, are appreciated for their salty bite and the simple way they enhance the flavor of pasta, baked fish, and sauces.

Canned tomatoes

Both fresh and canned tomatoes are common ingredients in the Mediterranean, whether they are used whole, diced, stewed, or condensed into a paste. Due to the heating process, tomato products in cans are particularly high in lycopene, which may offer some cancer protection. Shakshuka and stuffed tomatoes are two Mediterranean dishes that heavily feature tomatoes.

Greek yogurt and artisanal cheeses

Small servings of full-fat dairy products are encouraged as part of the Mediterranean diet, along with an abundance of fresh fruits, vegetables, and healthy grains. Yogurt is fermented and a great source of probiotics for the digestive system, in addition to adding extra protein to meals that emphasize plants. Instead of some of the more processed kinds that are frequently sold in the United States, this region focuses on historically cultured cheeses (made from milk and natural cultures).

Feta cheese frequently goes with stews and seafood dishes in addition to being a component of the traditional Greek salad. The hard texture of halloumi cheese, which makes it perfect for grilling and frying, is well known. Manchego can be baked into egg dishes, while harder cheeses like Pecorino Romano and Parmigiano-Reggiano are frequently grated into pasta.

Red wine

Mediterranean cuisine frequently includes wine as a side dish, but this is usually done in moderation (a 5-ounce pour is the standard). Antioxidant polyphenols and the flavonoid resveratrol, which are found in particular in red wine, may help raise HDL cholesterol and lower LDL cholesterol levels

Recommended wines to go with various Mediterranean dishes

It's summer, and it's BBQ time! But what wine goes with what kind of food? Here are some of our favorite wines to go with different kinds of Mediterranean dishes.

-Pair an herbaceous Sauvignon Blanc with a zesty tomato salad-

-A fruity, dry Rosé works well for a light pasta dish like salmon linguine in a cream sauce-

-Cabernet Sauvignon and Syrah are both bold enough to stand up to the rich flavors of lamb stew.

-Chardonnay, Pinot Gris and Pinot Grigio make great choices to pair with a classic Baked Chicken dish.

-For more lamb dishes you can try Blancs de Noir.

-A rich, smoky Zinfandel pairs well with grilled steak or lamb chops.

-Chianti is the ideal wine for a tomato based pasta dish like Spaghetti Aglio e Olio (Spaghetti with Garlic and Olive Oil).

30 days meal plan

Days	Breakfast	Lunch	Dinner	Dessert
1	Mediterranean Pita Breakfast	Brown Rice Pilaf with Golden Raisins	Turkey Burgers with Mango Salsa	Butter Pie
2	Hummus Deviled Egg	Chinese Soy Eggplant	One-Pan Tuscan Chicken	Homemade Spinach Pie
3	Smoked Salmon Scrambled Egg	Cauliflower Mash	Chicken Kapama	Rhubarb Strawberry Crunch
4	Buckwheat Apple-Raisin Muffin	Vegetarian Cabbage Rolls	Spinach and Feta–Stuffed Chicken Breasts	Banana Dessert with Chocolate Chips
5	Pumpkin Bran Muffin	Vegan Sesame Tofu and Eggplants	Rosemary Baked Chicken Drumsticks	Cranberry and Pistachio Biscotti
6	Buckwheat Buttermilk Pancakes	Steamed Squash Chowder	Chicken with Onions, Potatoes, Figs, and Carrots	Mascarpone and Fig Crostini
7	French Toast with Almonds and Peach Compote	Collard Green Wrap Greek Style	Moussaka	Crunchy Sesame Cookies
8	Mixed Berries Oatmeal with Sweet Vanilla Cream	Cayenne Eggplant Spread	Chicken in Tomato-Balsamic Pan Sauce	Almond Cookies
9	Choco-Strawberry Crepe	Cilantro Potato Mash	Seasoned Buttered Chicken	Baklava and Honey
10	No Crust Asparagus-Ham Quiche	Cheese and Broccoli Balls	Double Cheesy Bacon Chicken	Date and Nut Balls
11	Apple Cheese Scones	Hot Pepper Sauce	Chili Oregano Baked Cheese	Creamy Rice Pudding
12	Bacon and Egg Wrap	Avocado Gazpacho	Crispy Italian Chicken	Ricotta-Lemon Cheesecake
13	Orange-Blueberry Muffin	Roasted Garlic Hummus	Sea Bass in a Pocket	Crockpot Keto Chocolate Cake
14	Baked Ginger Oatmeal with Pear Topping	Pistachio-Crusted Whitefish	Creamy Smoked Salmon Pasta	Keto Crockpot Chocolate Lava Cake

15	Greek Style Veggie Omelet	Grilled Fish on Lemons	Slow Cooker Greek Chicken	Lemon Crockpot Cake
16	Summer Smoothie	Weeknight Sheet Pan Fish Dinner	Chicken Gyros	Lemon and Watermelon Granita
17	Ham & Egg Pitas	Crispy Polenta Fish Sticks	Slow Cooker Chicken Cassoulet	Baked Apples with Walnuts and Spices
18	Breakfast Couscous	Crispy Homemade Fish Sticks Recipe	Slow Cooker Chicken Provencal	Red Wine Poached Pears
19	Peach Breakfast Salad	Sauced Shellfish in White Wine	Greek Style Turkey Roast	Vanilla Pudding with Strawberries
20	Savory Oats	Pistachio Sole Fish	Garlic Chicken with Couscous	Mixed Berry Frozen Yogurt Bar
21	Tahini & Apple Toast	Speedy Tilapia with Red Onion and Avocado	Chicken Karahi	Fruit Salad with Yogurt Cream
22	Scrambled Basil Eggs	Tuscan Tuna and Zucchini Burgers	Chicken Cacciatore with Orzo	Date Nut Energy Balls
23	Greek Potatoes & Eggs	Sicilian Kale and Tuna Bowl	Tuscan Kale Salad with Anchovies	Pastaflora
24	Avocado & Honey Smoothie	Mediterranean Cod Stew	Peppers and Lentils Salad	Blueberry-Blackberry Ice Pops
25	Vegetable Frittata	Steamed Mussels in White Wine Sauce	Cashews and Red Cabbage Salad	Strawberry-Lime Ice Pops
26	Mini Lettuce Wraps	Orange and Garlic Shrimp	Tuscan Kale Salad with Anchovies	Coffee Ice Pops
27	Curry Apple Couscous	Roasted Shrimp-Gnocchi Bake	Apples and Pomegranate Salad	Fudge Ice Pops
28	Lamb & Vegetable Bake	Salmon Skillet Supper	Cranberry Bulgur Mix	Root Beer Float
29	Herb Flounder	Baked Cod with Vegetables	Chickpeas, Corn and Black Beans Salad	Orange Cream Float
30	Cauliflower Quinoa	Slow Cooker Salmon in Foil	Olives and Lentils Salad	Strawberry Shake

Breakfast and Smoothies Recipes

1. Mediterranean Pita Breakfast

Preparation Time: 22 minutes

Cooking Time: 3 minutes

Servings: 2

Ingredients:

- 1/4 cup of sweet red pepper
- 1/4 cup of chopped onion
- 1 cup of egg substitute
- 1/8 teaspoon of salt
- 1/8 teaspoon of pepper
- 1 small chopped tomato
- 1/2 cup of fresh torn baby spinach
- 1-1/2 teaspoons of minced fresh basil
- 2 whole size pita breads
- 2 tablespoons of crumbled feta cheese

Directions:

1. Coat with a cooking spray a small size non-stick skillet. Stir in the onion and red pepper for 3 minutes over medium heat. Add your egg substitute and season with salt and pepper. Stir cook until it sets. Mix the torn spinach, chopped tomatoes, and mince basil. Scoop onto the pitas. Top vegetable mixture with your egg mixture. Topped with crumbled feta cheese and serve immediately.

Nutrition (for 100g)

267 Calories

3g Fat

41g Carbohydrates

20g Protein

643mg Sodium

2. Hummus Deviled Egg

Preparation Time: 10 minutes

Cooking Time: 0 minute

Servings: 6

Ingredients:

- 1/4 cup of finely diced cucumber
- 1/4 cup of finely diced tomato
- 2 teaspoons of fresh lemon juice
- 1/8 teaspoon salt
- 6 hard-cooked peeled eggs, sliced half lengthwise
- 1/3 cup of roasted garlic hummus or any hummus flavor
- Chopped fresh parsley (optional)

Directions:

1. Combine the tomato, lemon juice, cucumber and salt together and then gently mix. Scrape out the yolks from the halved eggs and store for later use. Scoop a heaping teaspoon of humus in each half egg. Top with parsley and half-teaspoon tomato-cucumber mixture. Serve immediately

Nutrition (for 100g):

40 Calories

1g Fat

3g Carbohydrates

4g Protein

544mg Sodium

3. Smoked Salmon Scrambled Egg

Preparation Time: 2 minutes

Cooking Time: 8 minutes

Servings: 4

Ingredients:

- 16 ounces egg substitute, cholesterol-free
- 1/8 teaspoon of black pepper
- 2 tablespoons of sliced green onions, keep the tops
- 1 ounce of chilled reduced-fat cream cheese, cut into 1/4-inch cubes

- 2 ounces of flaked smoked salmon

Directions:

1. Cut the chilled cream cheese into ¼-inch cubes then set aside. Whisk the egg substitute and the pepper in a large sized bowl Coat a non-stick skillet with cooking spray over medium heat. Stir in the egg substitute and cook for 5 to 7 minutes or until it starts to set stirring occasionally and scraping bottom of the pan.

2. Fold in the cream cheese, green onions and the salmon. Continue to cook and stir for another 3 minutes or just until the eggs are still moist but cooked.

Nutrition (for 100g):

100 Calories

3g Fats

2g Carbohydrates

15g Protein

772mg Sodium

4. Buckwheat Apple-Raisin Muffin

Preparation Time: 24 minutes

Cooking Time: 20 minutes

Servings: 12

Ingredients:

- 1 cup of all-purpose flour
- 3/4 cup of buckwheat flour
- 2 tablespoons of brown sugar
- 1 1/2 teaspoons of baking powder
- 1/4 teaspoon of baking soda
- 3/4 cup of reduced-fat buttermilk
- 2 tablespoons of olive oil
- 1 large egg
- 1 cup peeled and cored, fresh diced apples
- 1/4 cup of golden raisins

Directions:

1. Prepare the oven at 375 degrees F. Line a 12-cup muffin tin with a non-stick cooking spray or paper cups. Set aside.

Incorporate all the dry ingredients in a mixing bowl. Set aside.

2. Beat together the liquid ingredients until smooth. Transfer the liquid mixture over the flour mixture and mix until moistened. Fold in the diced apples and raisins. Fill each muffin cups with about 2/3 full of the mixture. Bake until it turns golden brown. Use the toothpick test. Serve.

Nutrition (for 100g)

117 Calories

1g Fat

19g Carbohydrates

3g Protein

683mg Sodium

5. Pumpkin Bran Muffin

Preparation Time: 20 minutes

Cooking Time: 20 minutes

Servings: 22

Ingredients:

- 3/4 cup of all-purpose flour
- 3/4 cup of whole wheat flour
- 2 tablespoons sugar
- 1 tablespoon of baking powder
- 1/8 teaspoon salt
- 1 teaspoon of pumpkin pie spice
- 2 cups of 100% bran cereal
- 1 1/2 cups of skim milk
- 2 egg whites
- 15 ounces x 1 can pumpkin
- 2 tablespoons of avocado oil

Directions:

1. Preheat the oven to 400 degrees Fahrenheit. Prepare a muffin pan enough for 22 muffins and line with a non-stick cooking spray. Stir together the first four ingredients until combined. Set aside.

2. Using a large mixing bowl, mix together milk and cereal bran and let it stand for 2

minutes or until the cereal softens. Add in the oil, egg whites, and pumpkin in the bran mix and blend well. Fill in the flour mixture and mix well.

3. Divide the batter into equal portions into the muffin pan. Bake for 20 minutes. Pull out the muffins from pan and serve warm or cooled.

Nutrition (for 100g):

70 Calories

3g Fat

14g Carbohydrates

3g Protein

484mg Sodium

6. Buckwheat Buttermilk Pancakes

Preparation Time: 2 minutes

Cooking Time: 18 minutes

Servings: 9

Ingredients:

- 1/2 cup of buckwheat flour
- 1/2 cup of all-purpose flour
- 2 teaspoons of baking powder
- 1 teaspoon of brown sugar
- 2 tablespoons of olive oil
- 2 large eggs
- 1 cup of reduced-fat buttermilk

Directions:

1. Incorporate the first four ingredients in a bowl. Add the oil, buttermilk, and eggs and mix until thoroughly blended. Put griddle over medium heat and spray with non-stick cooking spray. Pour ¼ cup of the batter over the skillet and cook for 1-2 minutes each side or until they turn golden brown. Serve immediately.

Nutrition (for 100g)

108 Calories

3g Fat

12g Carbohydrates

4g Protein

556mg Sodium

7. French Toast with Almonds and Peach Compote

Preparation Time: 10 minutes

Cooking Time: 15 minutes

Servings: 4

Ingredients:

Compote:

- 3 tablespoons of sugar substitute, sucralose-based
- 1/3 cup + 2 tablespoons of water, divided
- 1 1/2 cups of fresh peeled or frozen, thawed and drained sliced peaches
- 2 tablespoons peach fruit spread, no-sugar-added
- 1/4 teaspoon of ground cinnamon
- Almond French toast
- 1/4 cup of (skim) fat-free milk
- 3 tablespoons of sugar substitute, sucralose-based
- 2 whole eggs
- 2 egg whites
- 1/2 teaspoon of almond extract
- 1/8 teaspoon salt
- 4 slices of multigrain bread
- 1/3 cup of sliced almonds

Directions:

1. To make the compote, dissolve 3 tablespoons sucralose in 1/3 cup of water in a medium saucepan over high-medium heat. Stir in the peaches and bring to a boil. Reduce the heat to medium and continue to cook uncovered for another 5 minutes or until the peaches softened.

2. Combine remaining water and fruit spread then stir into the peaches in the saucepan. Cook for another minute or until syrup thickens. Pull out from heat and add in the cinnamon. Cover to keep warm.

3. To make the French toast. Combine the milk and sucralose in a large size shallow dish and whisk until it completely dissolves. Whisk in the egg whites, eggs, almond extract and salt. Dip both sides of the bread slices for 3 minutes in the egg mixture or until completely soaked. Sprinkle both sides with sliced almonds and press firmly to adhere.

4. Brush the non-stick skillet with cooking spray and place over medium-high heat. Cook bread slices on griddle for 2 to 3 minutes both sides or until it turns light brown. Serve topped with the peach compote.

Nutrition (for 100g):

277 Calories

7g Fat

31g Carbohydrates

12g Protein

665mg Sodium

8. Mixed Berries Oatmeal with Sweet Vanilla Cream

Preparation Time: 5 minutes

Cooking Time: 5 minutes

Servings: 4

Ingredients:

- 2 cups water
- 1 cup of quick-cooking oats
- 1 tablespoon of sucralose-based sugar substitute
- 1/2 teaspoon of ground cinnamon
- 1/8 teaspoon salt
- Cream
- 3/4 cup of fat-free half-and-half
- 3 tablespoons of sucralose-based sugar substitute
- 1/2 teaspoon of vanilla extract
- 1/2 teaspoon of almond extract
- Toppings
- 1 1/2 cups of fresh blueberries

- 1/2 cup of fresh or frozen and thawed raspberries

Directions:

1. Boil water in high-heat and stir in the oats. Reduce heat to medium while cooking oats, uncovered for 2 minutes or until thick. Remove from heat and stir in sugar substitute, salt and cinnamon. In a medium size bowl, incorporate all the cream ingredients until well blended. Scoop cooked oatmeal into 4 equal portions and pour the sweet cream over. Top with the berries and serve.

Nutrition (for 100g):

150 Calories

5g Fat

30g Carbohydrates

5g Protein

807mg Sodium

9. Choco-Strawberry Crepe

Preparation Time: 5 minutes

Cooking Time: 10 minutes

Servings: 4

Ingredients:

- 1 cup of wheat all-purpose flour
- 2/3 cup of low-fat (1%) milk
- 2 egg whites
- 1 egg
- 3 tablespoons sugar
- 3 tablespoons of unsweetened cocoa powder
- 1 tablespoon of cooled melted butter
- 1/2 teaspoon salt
- 2 teaspoons of canola oil
- 3 tablespoons of strawberry fruit spread
- 3 1/2 cups of sliced thawed frozen or fresh strawberries
- 1/2 cup of fat-free thawed frozen whipped topping
- Fresh mint leaves (if desired)

Directions:

1. Incorporate the first eight ingredients in a large size bowl until smooth and thoroughly blended.
2. Brush ¼-teaspoon oil on a small size non-stick skillet over medium heat. Pour ¼-cup of the batter onto the center and swirl to coat the pan with batter.
3. Cook for a minute or until crêpe turns dull and the edges dry. Flip on the other side and cook for another half a minute. Repeat process with remaining mixture and oil.
4. Scoop ¼-cup of thawed strawberries at the center of the crepe and toll up to cover filling. Top with 2 tablespoons whipped cream and garnish with mint before serving.

Nutrition (for 100g):

334 Calories

5g Fat

58g Carbohydrates

10g Protein

678mg Sodium

10. No Crust Asparagus-Ham Quiche

Preparation Time: 5 minutes

Cooking Time: 42 minutes

Servings: 6

Ingredients:

- 2 cups 1/2-inched sliced asparagus
- 1 red chopped bell pepper
- 1 cup milk, low-fat (1%)
- 2 tablespoons of wheat all-purpose flour
- 4 egg whites
- 1 egg, whole
- 1 cup cooked chopped deli ham
- 2 tablespoons fresh chopped tarragon or basil
- 1/2 teaspoon of salt (optional)
- 1/4 teaspoon of black pepper
- 1/2 cup Swiss cheese, finely shredded

Directions:

1. Preheat your oven to 350 degrees F. Microwave bell pepper and asparagus in a tablespoon of water on HIGH for 2 minutes. Drain. Whisk flour and milk, and then add egg and egg whites until well combined. Stir in the vegetables and the remaining ingredients except the cheese.
2. Pour in a 9-inch size pie dish and bake for 35 minutes. Sprinkle cheese over the quiche and bake another 5 minutes or until cheese melts. Allow it cool for 5 minutes then cut into 6 wedges to serve.

Nutrition (for 100g):

138 Calories

1g Fat

8g Carbohydrates

13g Protein

588mg Sodium

11. Apple Cheese Scones

Preparation Time: 20 minutes

Cooking Time: 15 minutes

Servings: 10

Ingredients:

- 1 cup of all-purpose flour
- 1 cup whole wheat flour, white
- 3 tablespoons sugar
- 1 1/2 teaspoons of baking powder
- 1/2 teaspoon salt
- 1/2 teaspoon of ground cinnamon
- 1/4 teaspoon of baking soda
- 1 diced Granny Smith apple
- 1/2 cup shredded sharp Cheddar cheese
- 1/3 cup applesauce, natural or unsweetened
- 1/4 cup milk, fat-free (skim)
- 3 tablespoons of melted butter
- 1 egg

Directions:

1. Prepare your oven to 425 degrees F. Ready the baking sheet by lining with parchment paper. Merge all dry ingredients in a bowl and mix. Stir in the cheese and apple. Set aside. Whisk all the wet ingredients together. Pour over the dry mixture until blended and turns like a sticky dough.
2. Work on the dough on a floured surface about 5 times. Pat and then stretch into an 8-inch circle. Slice into 10 diagonal cuts.
3. Place on the baking sheet and spray top with cooking spray. Bake for 15 minutes or until lightly golden. Serve.

Nutrition (for 100g)

169 Calories

2g Fat

26g Carbohydrates

5g Protein

689mg Sodium

12. Bacon and Egg Wrap

Preparation Time: 15 minutes

Cooking Time: 15 minutes

Servings: 4

Ingredients:

- 1 cup egg substitute, cholesterol-free
- 1/4 cup Parmesan cheese, shredded
- 2 slices diced Canadian bacon
- 1/2 teaspoon red hot pepper sauce
- 1/4 teaspoon of black pepper
- 4x7-inch whole wheat tortillas
- 1 cup of baby spinach leaves

Directions:

1. Preheat your oven at 325 degrees F. Combine the first five ingredients to make the filling. Pour the mixture in a 9-inch glass dish sprayed with butter-flavored cooking spray.

2. Bake for 15 minutes or until egg sets. Remove from oven. Place the tortillas for a minute in the oven. Cut baked egg mixture into quarters. Arrange one quarter at the center of each tortillas and top with ¼-cup spinach. Fold tortilla from the bottom to the center and then both sides to the center to enclose. Serve immediately.

Nutrition (for 100g):

195 Calories

3g Fat

20g Carbohydrates

15g Protein

688mg Sodium

13. Orange-Blueberry Muffin

Preparation Time: 10 minutes

Cooking Time: 20 - 25 minutes

Servings: 12

Ingredients:

- 1 3/4 cups of all-purpose flour
- 1/3 cup sugar
- 2 1/2 teaspoons of baking powder
- 1/2 teaspoon of baking soda
- 1/2 teaspoon salt
- 1/2 teaspoon of ground cinnamon
- 3/4 cup milk, fat-free (skim)
- 1/4 cup butter
- 1 egg, large, lightly beaten
- 3 tablespoons thawed orange juice concentrate
- 1 teaspoon vanilla
- 3/4 cup fresh blueberries

Directions:

1. Ready your oven to 400 degrees F. Follow steps 2 to 5 of Buckwheat Apple-Raisin Muffin Fill up the muffin cups ¾-full of the mixture and bake for 20 to 25 minutes. Let it cool 5 minutes and serve warm.

Nutrition (for 100g)

149 Calories

5g Fat

24g Carbohydrates

3g Protein

518mg Sodium

14. Baked Ginger Oatmeal with Pear Topping

Preparation Time: 10 minutes

Cooking Time: 15 minutes

Servings: 2

Ingredients:

- 1 cup of old-fashioned oats
- 3/4 cup milk, fat-free (skim)
- 1 egg white
- 1 1/2 teaspoons grated ginger, fresh or 3/4 teaspoon of ground ginger
- 2 tablespoons brown sugar, divided
- 1/2 ripe diced pear

Directions:

1. Spray 2x6 ounce ramekins with a non-stick cooking spray. Prepare the oven to 350 degrees F. Combine the first four ingredients and a tablespoon of sugar then mix well. Pour evenly between the 2 ramekins. Top with pear slices and the remaining tablespoon of sugar. Bake for 15 minutes. Serve warm.

Nutrition (for 100g)

268 Calories

5g fat

2g Carbohydrates

10g Protein

779mg Sodium

15. Greek Style Veggie Omelet

Preparation Time: 10 minutes

Cooking Time: 20 minutes

Servings: 2

Ingredients:

- 4 large eggs
- 2 tablespoons of fat-free milk
- 1/8 teaspoon salt
- 3 teaspoons of olive oil, divided
- 2 cups baby Portobello, sliced
- 1/4 cup of finely chopped onion
- 1 cup of fresh baby spinach
- 3 tablespoons feta cheese, crumbled
- 2 tablespoons ripe olives, sliced
- Freshly ground pepper

Directions:

1. Whisk together first three ingredients. Stir in 2 tablespoons of oil in a non-stick skillet over medium-high heat. Sauté the onions and mushroom for 5-6 minutes or until golden brown. Mix in the spinach and cook. Remove mixture from pan.
2. Using the same pan, heat over medium-low heat the remaining oil. Pour your egg mixture and as it starts to set, pushed the edges towards the center to let the uncooked mixture flow underneath. When eggs set scoop the veggie mixture on one side. Sprinkle with olives and feta then fold the other side to close. Slice in half and sprinkle with pepper to serve.

Nutrition (for 100g)

271 Calories

2g Fat

7g Carbohydrates

18g Protein

648mg Sodium

16. Summer Smoothie

Preparation Time: 8 minutes

Cooking Time: 0 minute

Servings: 2

Ingredients:

- 1/2 Banana, Peeled
- 2 Cups Strawberries, Halved
- 3 Tablespoons Mint, Chopped
- 1 1/2 Cups Coconut Water
- 1/2 Avocado, Pitted & Peeled
- 1 Date, Chopped
- Ice Cubes as Needed

Directions:

1. Incorporate everything in a blender, and process until smooth. Add ice cubes to thicken, and serve chilled.

Nutrition (for 100g):

360 calories

12g fats

5g carbohydrates

31g protein

737mg sodium

17. Ham & Egg Pitas

Preparation Time: 5 minutes

Cooking Time: 15 minutes

Servings: 4

Ingredients:

- 6 Eggs
- 2 Shallots, Chopped
- 1 Teaspoon Olive Oil
- 1/3 Cup Smoked Ham, Chopped
- 1/3 Cup Sweet Green Pepper, Chopped
- 1/4 Cup Brie Cheese
- Sea Salt & Black Pepper to Taste
- 4 Lettuce Leaves
- 2 Pita Breads, Whole Wheat

Directions:

1. Heat the olive oil in a pan using medium heat. Add in your shallots and green pepper, letting them cook for five minutes while stirring frequently.
2. Get out a bowl and whip your eggs, sprinkling in your salt and pepper. Make sure your eggs are well beaten. Put the eggs into the pan, and then mix in the ham and cheese. Stir well, and cook until your mixture thickens. Split the pitas in half, and open the pockets. Spread a teaspoon of mustard in each pocket, and add a lettuce leaf in each one. Spread the egg mixture in each one and serve.

Nutrition (for 100g):

610 calories

21g fats

10g carbohydrates

41g protein

807mg sodium

18. Breakfast Couscous

Preparation Time: 5 minutes

Cooking Time: 15 minutes

Servings: 4

Ingredients:

- 3 Cups Milk, Low Fat
- 1 Cinnamon Stick
- 1/2 Cup Apricots, Dried & Chopped
- 1/4 Cup Currants, Dried
- 1 Cup Couscous, Uncooked
- Pinch Sea Salt, Fine
- 4 Teaspoons Butter, Melted
- 6 Teaspoons Brown Sugar

Directions:

1. Heat a pan up with milk and cinnamon using medium-high heat. Cook for three minutes before removing the pan from heat.
2. Add in your apricots, couscous, salt, currants, and sugar. Stir well, and then

cover. Leave it to the side, and let it sit for fifteen minutes.

Throw out the cinnamon stick, and divide between bowls. Sprinkle with brown sugar before serving.

Nutrition (for 100g):

520 calories

28g fats

10g carbohydrates

39g protein

619mg sodium

19. Peach Breakfast Salad

Preparation Time: 10 minutes

Cooking Time: 0 minute

Servings: 1

Ingredients:

- 1/4 Cup Walnuts, Chopped & Toasted
- 1 Teaspoon Honey, Raw
- 1 Peach, Pitted & Sliced
- 1/2 Cup Cottage Cheese, Nonfat & Room Temperature
- 1 Tablespoon Mint, Fresh & Chopped
- 1 Lemon, Zested

Directions:

1. Place your cottage cheese in a bowl, and top with peach slices and walnuts. Drizzle with honey, and top with mint.
2. Sprinkle on your lemon zest before serving immediately.

Nutrition (for 100g):

280 calories

11g fats

19g carbohydrates

39g protein

527mg sodium

20. Savory Oats

Preparation Time: 10 minutes

Cooking Time: 10 minutes

Servings: 2

Ingredients:

- 1/2 Cup Steel Cut Oats
- 1 Cup Water
- 1 Tomato, Large & Chopped
- 1 Cucumber, Chopped
- 1 Tablespoon Olive Oil
- Sea Salt & Black Pepper to Taste
- Flat Leaf Parsley, Chopped to Garnish
- Parmesan Cheese, Low Fat & Freshly Grated

Directions:

1. Bring your oats and a cup of water to a boil using a saucepan over high heat. Stir often until your water is completely absorbed, which will take roughly fifteen minutes. Divide between two bowls, and top with tomatoes and cucumber. Drizzle with olive oil and top with parmesan. Garnish with parsley before serving.

Nutrition (for 100g):

408 calories

13g fats

10g carbohydrates

28g protein

825mg sodium

21. Tahini & Apple Toast

Preparation Time: 15 minutes

Cooking Time: 0 minute

Servings: 1

Ingredients:

- 2 Tablespoons Tahini
- 2 Slices Whole Wheat Bread, Toasted
- 1 Teaspoon Honey, Raw

- 1 Apple, Small, Cored & Sliced Thin

Directions:

1. Start by spreading the tahini over your toast, and then lay your apples over it. drizzle with honey before serving.

Nutrition (for 100g):

366 calories

13g fats

9g carbohydrates

29g protein

686mg sodium

22. Scrambled Basil Eggs

Preparation Time: 5 minutes

Cooking Time: 10 minutes

Servings: 2

Ingredients:

- 4 Eggs, Large
- 2 Tablespoons Fresh Basil, Chopped Fine
- 2 Tablespoons Gruyere Cheese, Grated
- 1 Tablespoon Cream
- 1 Tablespoon Olive Oil
- 2 Cloves Garlic, Minced
- Sea Salt & Black Pepper to Taste

Directions:

1. Get out a large bowl and beat your basil, cheese, cream and eggs together. Whisk until it's well combined. Get out a large skillet over medium-low heat, and heat your oil. Add in your garlic, cooking for a minute. It should turn golden.
2. Pour the egg mixture into your skillet over the garlic, and then continue to scramble as they cook so they become soft and fluffy. Season it well and serve warm.

Nutrition (for 100g):

360 calories

14g fats

8g carbohydrates

29g protein

545mg sodium

23. Greek Potatoes & Eggs

Preparation Time: 10 minutes

Cooking Time: 30 minutes

Servings: 2

Ingredients:

- 3 tomatoes, seeded & roughly chopped
- 2 tablespoons basil, fresh & chopped
- 1 clove garlic, minced
- 2 tablespoons + ½ cup olive oil, divided
- sea salt & black pepper to taste
- 3 russet potatoes, large
- 4 eggs, large
- 1 teaspoon oregano, fresh & chopped

Directions:

1. Get the food processor and place your tomatoes in, pureeing them with the skin on.
2. Add your garlic, two tablespoons of oil, salt, pepper and basil. Pulse until it's well combined. Place this mixture in a skillet, cooking while covered for twenty to twenty-five minutes over low heat. Your sauce should be thickened as well as bubbly.
3. Dice your potatoes into cubes, and then place them in a skillet with a ½ a cup of olive oil in a skillet using medium-low heat.
4. Fry your potatoes until crisp and browned. This should take five minutes, and then cover the skillet, reducing the heat to low. Steam them until your potatoes are done.
5. Stir in the eggs into the tomato sauce, and cook using low heat for six minutes. Your eggs should be set.
6. Remove the potatoes from your pan, and drain using paper towels. Place them in a bowl. Sprinkle in your salt, pepper and

oregano, and then serve your eggs with potatoes. Drizzle your sauce over the mixture, and serve warm.

Nutrition (for 100g):

348 calories

12g fats

7g carbohydrates

27g protein

469mg sodium

24. Avocado & Honey Smoothie

Preparation Time: 5 minutes

Cooking Time: 0 minute

Servings: 2

Ingredients:

- 1 1/2 cups soy milk
- 1 avocado, large
- 2 tablespoons honey, raw

Directions:

1. Incorporate all ingredients together and blend until smooth, and serve immediately.

Nutrition (for 100g):

280 calories

19g fats

11g carbohydrates

30g protein

547mg sodium

25. Vegetable Frittata

Preparation Time: 5 minutes

Cooking Time: 10 minutes

Servings: 2

Ingredients:

- 1/2 baby eggplant, peeled & diced
- 1 handful baby spinach leaves
- 1 tablespoon olive oil
- 3 eggs, large
- 1 teaspoon almond milk
- 1-ounce goat cheese, crumbled
- 1/4 small red pepper, chopped
- sea salt & black pepper to taste

Directions:

2. Start by heating the broiler on your oven, and then beat the eggs together with almond milk. Make sure it's well combined, and then get out a nonstick, oven proof skillet. Place it over medium-high heat, and then add in your olive oil.
3. Once your oil is heated, add in your eggs. Spread your spinach over this mixture in an even layer, and top with the rest of your vegetables.
4. Reduce your heat to medium, and sprinkle with salt and pepper. Allow your vegetables and eggs to cook for five minutes. The bottom half of your eggs should be firm, and your vegetables should be tender. Top with goat cheese, and then broil on the middle rack for three to five minutes. Your eggs should be all the way done, and your cheese should be melted. Slice into wedges and serve warm.

Nutrition (for 100g):

340 calories

16g fats

9g carbohydrates

37g protein

748mg sodium

26. Mini Lettuce Wraps

Preparation Time: 15 minutes

Cooking Time: 0 minute

Servings: 4

Ingredients:

- 1 cucumber, diced
- 1 red onion, sliced
- 1-ounce feta cheese, low fat & crumbed
- 1 lemon, juiced
- 1 tomato, diced
- 1 tablespoon olive oil
- 12 small iceberg lettuce leaves
- sea salt & black pepper to taste

Directions:

1. Combine your tomato, onion, feta, and cucumber together in a bowl. Mix your oil and juice, and season with salt and pepper.
2. Fill each leaf with the vegetable mixture, and roll them tightly. Use a toothpick to keep them together to serve.

Nutrition (for 100g):

291 calories

10g fats

9g carbohydrates

27g protein

655mg sodium

27. Curry Apple Couscous

Preparation Time: 20 minutes

Cooking Time: 5 minutes

Servings: 4

Ingredients:

- 2 teaspoons olive oil
- 2 leeks, white parts only, sliced
- 1 apple, diced
- 2 tablespoons curry powder
- 2 cups couscous, cooked & whole wheat
- 1/2 cup pecans, chopped

Directions:

1. Heat your oil in a skillet using medium heat. Add the leeks, and cook until tender, which will take five minutes. Add in your apple, and cook until soft.
2. Add in your curry powder and couscous, and stir well. Remove from heat, and mix in your nuts before serving immediately.

Nutrition (for 100g):

330 calories

12g fats

8g carbohydrates

30g protein

824mg sodium

28. Lamb & Vegetable Bake

Preparation Time: 20 minutes

Cooking Time: 1 hour and 10 minutes

Servings: 8

Ingredients:

- 1/4 cup olive oil
- 1 lb. lean lamb, boneless & chopped into ½ inch pieces
- 2 red potatoes, large, scrubbed & diced
- 1 onion, chopped roughly
- 2 cloves garlic, minced
- 28 ounces diced tomatoes with liquid, canned & no salt
- 2 zucchinis, cut into ½ inch slices
- 1 red bell pepper, seeded & cut into 1-inch cubes
- 2 tablespoons flat leaf parsley, chopped
- 1 tablespoon paprika
- 1 teaspoon thyme
- 1/2 teaspoon cinnamon
- 1/2 cup red wine
- sea salt & black pepper to taste

Directions:

1. Start by turning the oven to 325, and then get out a large stew pot. Place it over medium-high heat to heat your olive oil. Once your oil is hot stir in your lamb, browning the meat. Stir frequently to keep it from running, and then place your

lamb in a baking dish. Cook your garlic, onion and potatoes in the skillet until they're tender, which should take five to six minutes more. Place them to the baking dish as well. Pour the zucchini, pepper, and tomatoes in the pan with your herbs and spices. Allow it to simmer for ten minutes more before pouring it into your baking dish. Pour in the wine and pepper sauce. Add in your tomato, and then cover with foil. Bake for an hour. Take the cover off for the last fifteen minutes of baking, and adjust seasoning as needed.

Nutrition (for 100g):

240 calories

14g fats

8g carbohydrates

36g protein

427mg sodium

29. Herb Flounder

Preparation Time: 20 minutes

Cooking Time: 1 hour and 5 minutes

Servings: 4

Ingredients:

- 1/2 cup flatleaf parsley, lightly packed
- 1/4 cup olive oil
- 4 cloves garlic, peeled & halved
- 2 tablespoons rosemary, fresh
- 2 tablespoons thyme leaves, fresh
- 2 tablespoons sage, fresh
- 2 tablespoons lemon zest, fresh
- 4 flounder fillets
- sea salt & black pepper to taste

Directions:

2. Ready your oven to 350, and then put all of the ingredients except for the flounder in the processor. Blend until it forms at hick paste. Put your fillets on a baking sheet, and brush them down with the paste. Allow them to chill in the fridge for

an hour. Bake for ten minutes. Season and serve warm.

Nutrition (for 100g):

307 calories

11g fats

7g carbohydrates

34g protein

824mg sodium

30. Cauliflower Quinoa

Preparation Time: 15 minutes

Cooking Time: 10 minutes

Servings: 4

Ingredients:

- 1 1/2 cups quinoa, cooked
- 3 tablespoons olive oil
- 3 cups cauliflower florets
- 2 spring onions, chopped
- 1 tablespoon red wine vinegar
- sea salt & black pepper to taste
- 1 tablespoon red wine vinegar
- 1 tablespoon chives, chopped
- 1 tablespoon parsley, chopped

Directions:

1. Start by heating up a pan over medium-high heat. Add your oil. Once your oil is hot, add in your spring onions and cook for about two minutes. Add in your quinoa and cauliflower, and then add in the rest of the ingredients. Mix well, and cover. Cook for nine minutes over medium heat, and divide between plates to serve.

Nutrition (for 100g):

290 calories

14g fats

9g carbohydrates

26g protein

656mg sodium

31. Mango Pear Smoothie

Preparation Time: 5 minutes

Cooking Time: 0 minute

Servings: 1

Ingredients:

- 2 ice cubes
- ½ cup Greek yogurt, plain
- ½ mango, peeled, pitted & chopped
- 1 cup kale, chopped
- 1 pear, ripe, cored & chopped

Directions:

1. Blend together until thick and smooth. Serve chilled.

Nutrition (for 100g):

350 calories

12g fats

9g carbohydrates

40g protein

457mg sodium

32. Spinach Omelet

Preparation Time: 10 minutes

Cooking Time: 20 minutes

Servings: 4

Ingredients:

- 3 tablespoons olive oil
- 1 onion, small & chopped
- 1 clove garlic, minced
- 4 tomatoes, large, cored & chopped
- 1 teaspoon sea salt, fine
- 8 eggs, beaten
- ¼ teaspoon black pepper
- 2 ounces feta cheese, crumbled
- 1 tablespoon flat leaf parsley, fresh & chopped

Directions:

2. Preheat oven to 400 degrees, and pour olive oil in an ovenproof skillet. Place your skillet over high heat, adding in your onions. Cook for five to seven minutes. Your onions should soften.
3. Add your tomatoes, salt, pepper and garlic in. Then simmer for another five minutes, and fill in your beaten eggs. Mix lightly, and cook for three to five minutes. They should set at the bottom. Put the pan in the oven, baking for five minutes more. Remove from the oven, topping with parsley and feta. Serve warm.

Nutrition (for 100g):

280 calories

19g fats

10g carbohydrates

31g protein

625mg sodium

33. Almond Pancakes

Preparation Time: 15 minutes

Cooking Time: 15 minutes

Servings: 6

Ingredients:

- 2 cups almond milk, unsweetened & room temperature
- 2 eggs, large & room temperature
- ½ cup coconut oil, melted + more for greasing
- 2 teaspoons honey, raw
- ¼ teaspoon sea salt, fine
- ½ teaspoon baking soda
- 1 ½ cups whole wheat flour
- ½ cup almond flour
- 1 ½ teaspoons baking powder
- ¼ teaspoon cinnamon, ground

Directions:

1. Get out a large bowl and whisk your coconut oil, eggs, almond milk and honey, blending until it's mixed well.
2. Get a medium bowl out and sift together your baking powder, baking soda, almond flour, sea salt, whole wheat flour and cinnamon. Mix well.
3. Add your flour mixture to your milk mixture, and whisk well.
4. Get out a large skillet and grease it using your coconut oil before placing it over medium-high heat. Add in your pancake batter in ½ cup measurements.
5. Cook for three minutes or until the edges are firm. The bottom of your pancake should be golden, and bubbles should break the surface. Cook both sides.
6. Wipe clean your skillet, and repeat until all of your batter is used. Make sure to re-grease your skillet, and top with fresh fruit if desired.

Nutrition (for 100g):

205 calories

16g fats

9g carbohydrates

36g protein

828mg sodium

34. Quinoa Fruit Salad

Preparation Time: 25 minutes

Cooking Time: 0 minute

Servings: 4

Ingredients:

- 2 tablespoons honey, raw
- 1 cup strawberries, fresh & sliced
- 2 tablespoons lime juice, fresh
- 1 teaspoon basil, fresh & chopped
- 1 cup quinoa, cooked
- 1 mango, peeled, pitted & diced
- 1 cup blackberries, fresh
- 1 peach, pitted & diced

- 2 kiwis, peeled & quartered

Directions:

1. Start by mixing your lime juice, basil and honey together in a small bowl. In a different bowl mix your strawberries, quinoa, blackberries, peach, kiwis and mango. Add in your honey mixture, and toss to coat before serving.

Nutrition (for 100g):

159 calories

12g fats

9g carbohydrates

29g protein

829mg sodium

35. Strawberry Rhubarb Smoothie

Preparation Time: 8 minutes

Cooking Time: 0 minute

Servings: 1

Ingredients:

- 1 cup strawberries, fresh & sliced
- 1 rhubarb stalk, chopped
- 2 tablespoons honey, raw
- 3 ice cubes
- 1/8 teaspoon ground cinnamon
- ½ cup Greek yogurt, plain

Directions:

2. Start by getting out a small saucepan and fill it with water. Place it over high heat to bring it to a boil, and then add in your rhubarb. Boil for three minutes before draining and transferring it to a blender.
3. In your blender add in your yogurt, honey, cinnamon and strawberries. Once smooth, stir in your ice. Blend until there are no lumps and it's thick. Enjoy cold.

Nutrition (for 100g):

201 calories

11g fats

9g carbohydrates

39g protein

657mg sodium

36. Barley Porridge

Preparation Time: 10 minutes

Cooking Time: 20 minutes

Servings: 4

Ingredients:

- 1 cup wheat berries
- 1 cup barley
- 2 cups almond milk, unsweetened + more for serving
- ½ cup blueberries
- ½ cup pomegranate seeds
- 2 cups water
- ½ cup hazelnuts, toasted & chopped
- ¼ cup honey, raw

Directions:

1. Get out a saucepan and put it over medium-high heat, and then add in your almond milk, water, barley and wheat berries. Let it boil before lowering the heat and allow it to simmer for twenty-five minutes. Stir frequently. Your grains should become tender.
2. Top each serving with blueberries, pomegranate seeds, hazelnuts, a tablespoon of honey and a splash of almond milk.

Nutrition (for 100g):

150 calories

10g fats

9g carbohydrates

29g protein

546mg sodium

37. Gingerbread & Pumpkin Smoothie

Preparation Time: 15 minutes

Cooking Time: 50 minutes

Servings: 1

Ingredients:

- 1 cup almond milk, unsweetened
- 2 teaspoons chia seeds
- 1 banana
- ½ cup pumpkin puree, canned
- ¼ teaspoon ginger, ground
- ¼ teaspoon cinnamon, ground
- 1/8 teaspoon nutmeg, ground

Directions:

1. Start by getting out a bowl and mix your chai seeds and almond milk. Allow them to soak for at least an hour, but you can soak them overnight. Transfer them to a blender.
2. Add in your remaining ingredients, and then blend until smooth. Serve chilled.

Nutrition (for 100g):

250 calories

13g fats

7g carbohydrates

26g protein

621mg sodium

38. Green Juice

Preparation Time: 5 minutes

Cooking Time: 0 minute

Servings: 1

Ingredients

- 3 cups dark leafy greens
- 1 cucumber
- ¼ cup fresh Italian parsley leaves
- ¼ pineapple, cut into wedges
- ½ green apple
- ½ orange
- ½ lemon
- Pinch grated fresh ginger

Directions

1. Using a juicer, run the greens, cucumber, parsley, pineapple, apple, orange, lemon, and ginger through it, pour into a large cup, and serve.

Nutrition (for 100g):

200 calories

14g fats

6g carbohydrates

27g protein

541mg sodium

39. Walnut & Date Smoothie

Preparation Time: 10 minutes

Cooking Time: 0 minute

Servings: 2

Ingredients:

- 4 dates, pitted
- ½ cup milk
- 2 cups Greek yogurt, plain
- 1/2 cup walnuts
- ½ teaspoon cinnamon, ground
- ½ teaspoon vanilla extract, pure
- 2-3 ice cubes

Directions:

1. Blend everything together until smooth, and then serve chilled.

Nutrition (for 100g):

109 calories

11g fats

7g carbohydrates

29g protein

732mg sodium

40. Fruit Smoothie

Preparation Time: 5 minutes

Cooking Time: 0 minute

Servings: 2

Ingredients

- 2 cups blueberries
- 2 cups unsweetened almond milk
- 1 cup crushed ice
- ½ teaspoon ground ginger

Directions

1. Put the blueberries, almond milk, ice, and ginger in a blender. Process until smooth.

Nutrition (for 100g):

115 calories

10g fats

5g carbohydrates

27g protein

912mg sodium

41. Chocolate Banana Smoothie

Preparation Time: 5 minutes

Cooking Time: 0 minute

Servings: 2

Ingredients

- 2 bananas, peeled
- 1 cup skim milk
- 1 cup crushed ice
- 3 tablespoons unsweetened cocoa powder
- 3 tablespoons honey

Directions

1. In a blender, mix the bananas, almond milk, ice, cocoa powder, and honey. Blend until smooth.

Nutrition (for 100g):

150 calories

18g fats

6g carbohydrates

30g protein

821mg sodium

42. Yogurt with Blueberries, Honey, and Mint

Preparation Time: 5 minutes

Cooking Time: 0 minute

Servings: 2

Ingredients

- 2 cups unsweetened nonfat plain Greek yogurt
- 1 cup blueberries
- 3 tablespoons honey
- 2 tablespoons fresh mint leaves, chopped

Directions

1. Apportion the yogurt between 2 small bowls. Top with the blueberries, honey, and mint.

Nutrition (for 100g):

126 calories

12g fats

8g carbohydrates

37g protein

932mg sodium

43. Berry and Yogurt Parfait

Preparation Time: 5 minutes

Cooking Time: 0 minute

Servings: 2

Ingredients

- 1 cup raspberries
- 1½ cups unsweetened nonfat plain Greek yogurt
- 1 cup blackberries
- ¼ cup chopped walnuts

Directions

1. In 2 bowls, layer the raspberries, yogurt, and blackberries. Sprinkle with the walnuts.

Nutrition (for 100g):

119 calories

13g fats

7g carbohydrates

28g protein

732mg sodium

44. Oatmeal with Berries and Sunflower Seeds

Preparation Time: 5 minutes

Cooking Time: 10 minutes

Servings: 4

Ingredients

- 1¾ cups water
- ½ cup unsweetened almond milk
- Pinch sea salt
- 1 cup old-fashioned oats
- ½ cup blueberries
- ½ cup raspberries
- ¼ cup sunflower seeds

Directions

2. Boil water with almond milk, and sea salt in a medium saucepan over medium-high heat.
3. Stir in the oats. Decrease the heat to medium-low and continue stirring and cook, for 5 minutes. Cover, and let the oatmeal stand for 2 minutes more. Stir and serve topped with the blueberries, raspberries, and sunflower seeds.

Nutrition (for 100g):

106 calories

9g fats

8g carbohydrates

29g protein

823mg sodium

45. Almond and Maple Quick Grits

Preparation Time: 5 minutes

Cooking Time: 10 minutes

Servings: 4

Ingredients

- 1½ cups water
- ½ cup unsweetened almond milk
- Pinch sea salt
- ½ cup quick-cooking grits
- ½ teaspoon ground cinnamon
- ¼ cup pure maple syrup
- ¼ cup slivered almonds

Directions

1. Put water, almond milk, and sea salt in a medium saucepan over medium-high heat and wait to boil.
2. Stir continuously with a wooden spoon, slowly add the grits. Continue stirring to prevent lumps and bring the mixture to a slow boil. Reduce the heat to medium-low. Simmer for few minutes, stirring regularly, until the water is completely absorbed.
3. Stir in the cinnamon, syrup, and almonds. Cook for 1 minute more, stirring.

Nutrition (for 100g):

126 calories

10g fats

7g carbohydrates

28g protein

851mg sodium

46. Banana Oats

Preparation Time: 10 minutes

Cooking Time: 10 minutes

Servings: 2

Ingredients

- 1 banana, peeled and sliced
- ¾ c. almond milk
- ½ c. cold-brewed coffee
- 2 pitted dates
- 2 tbsps. cocoa powder
- 1 c. rolled oats
- 1 ½ tbsps. chia seeds

Directions:

1. Using a blender, add in all ingredients. Process well for 5 minutes and serve.

Nutrition (for 100g):

288 Calories

4.4g Fat

10g Carbohydrates

5.9g Protein

733mg Sodium

47. Breakfast Sandwich

Preparation Time: 5 minutes

Cooking Time: 20 minutes

Servings: 4

Ingredients

- 4 multigrain sandwich thins
- 4 tsps. olive oil
- 4 eggs
- 1 tbsp. rosemary, fresh
- 2 c. baby spinach leaves, fresh
- 1 tomato, sliced
- 1 tbsp. of feta cheese
- Pinch of kosher salt
- Ground black pepper

Directions:

2. Prepare oven at 375 F/190 C. Brush the thins' sides with 2 tsps. of olive oil and set on a baking sheet. Set in the oven and toast for 5 minutes or until the edges are lightly brown.
3. In a skillet, add in the rest of the olive oil and rosemary to heat over high heat.

Break and place whole eggs one at a time into the skillet. The yolk should still be runny, but the egg whites should be set.

4. Break yolks up with a spatula. Flip the egg and cook on another side until done. Remove eggs from heat. Place toasted sandwich thins on 4 separate plates. Divine spinach among the thins.

5. Top each thin with two tomato slices, cooked egg, and 1 tbsp. of feta cheese. Lightly sprinkle with salt and pepper for flavoring. Place remaining sandwich thin halves over the top and they are ready to serve.

Nutrition (for 100g):

241 Calories

12.2g Fat

60.2g Carbohydrates

21g Protein

855mg Sodium

48. Morning Couscous

Preparation Time: 10 minutes

Cooking Time: 8 minutes

Servings: 4

Ingredients

- 3 c. low-fat milk
- 1 c. whole-wheat couscous, uncooked
- 1 cinnamon stick
- ½ chopped apricot, dried
- ¼ c. currants, dried
- 6 tsps. brown sugar
- ¼ tsp. salt
- 4 tsps. melted butter

Directions:

1. Take a large saucepan and combine milk and cinnamon stick and heat over medium. Heat for 3 minutes or until microbubbles forms around edges of the pan. Do not boil. Remove from heat, stir in the couscous, apricots, currants, salt, and 4 tsps. brown sugar. Cover the

mixture and allow it to sit for 15 minutes. Remove and throw away the cinnamon stick. Divide couscous among 4 bowls, and top each with 1 tsp. melted butter and ½ tsp. brown sugar. Ready to serve.

Nutrition (for 100g):

306 Calories

6g Fat

5g Carbohydrates

9g Protein

944mg Sodium

49. Avocado and Apple Smoothie

Preparation Time: 5 minutes

Cooking Time: 0 minute

Servings: 2

Ingredient

- 3 c. spinach
- 1 cored green apple, chopped
- 1 pitted avocado, peeled and chopped
- 3 tbsps. chia seeds
- 1 tsp. honey
- 1 frozen banana, peeled
- 2 c. coconut water

Directions:

1. Using your blender, add in all the ingredients. Process well for 5 minutes to obtain a smooth consistency and serve in glasses.

Nutrition (for 100g):

208 Calories

10.1g Fat

6g Carbohydrates

7g Protein

924mg Sodium

50. Mini Frittatas

Preparation Time: 10 minutes

Cooking Time: 20 minutes

Servings: 8

Ingredients

- 1 chopped yellow onion
- 1 c. grated parmesan
- 1 chopped yellow bell pepper
- 1 chopped red bell pepper
- 1 chopped zucchini
- Salt and black pepper
- A drizzle of olive oil
- 8 whisked eggs
- 2 tbsps. chopped chives

Directions:

2. Set a pan over medium-high heat. Add in oil to warm. Stir in all ingredients except chives and eggs. Sauté for around 5 minutes.
3. Put the eggs on a muffin pan and top by the chives. Set oven to 350 F/176 C. Place the muffin pans into the oven to bake for about 10 minutes. Serve the eggs on a plate with sautéed vegetables.

Nutrition (for 100g):

55 Calories

3g Fat

0.7g Carbohydrates

9g Protein

844mg Sodium

51. Sun-dried Tomatoes Oatmeal

Preparation Time: 10 minutes

Cooking Time: 25 minutes

Servings: 4

Ingredients

- 3 c. water
- 1 c. almond milk
- 1 tbsp. olive oil
- 1 c. steel-cut oats
- ¼ c. chopped tomatoes, sun-dried
- A pinch of red pepper flakes

Directions:

1. Using a pan, add water and milk to mix. Set on medium heat and allow to boil. Set up another pan on medium-high heat. Warm oil and add oats to cook for 2 minutes. Transfer to the first pan plus tomatoes then stir. Let simmer for approximately 20 minutes. Set in serving bowls and top with red pepper flakes. Enjoy.

Nutrition (for 100g):

170 Calories

17.8g Fat

1.5g Carbohydrates

10g Protein

645mg Sodium

52. Breakfast Egg on Avocado

Preparation Time: 5 minutes

Cooking Time: 15 minutes

Servings: 6

Ingredients

- 1 tsp. garlic powder
- ½ tsp. sea salt
- ¼ c. shredded Parmesan cheese
- ¼ tsp. black pepper
- 3 pitted avocados, halved
- 6 eggs

Directions:

2. Ready the muffin tins and prepare the oven at 350 F/176 C. Split the avocado. To ensure that the egg would fit inside the cavity of the avocado, lightly scrape off 1/3 of the meat.
3. Place avocado on a muffin tin to ensure that it faces with the top-up. Evenly

season each avocado with pepper, salt, and garlic powder. Add one egg on each avocado cavity and garnish tops with cheese. Set in your oven to bake until the egg white is set, about 15 minutes. Serve and enjoy.

Nutrition (for 100g):

252 Calories

20g Fat

2g Carbohydrates

5g Protein

946mg Sodium

53. Brekky Egg- Potato Hash

Preparation Time: 10 minutes

Cooking Time: 25 minutes

Servings: 2

Ingredients

- 1 zucchini, diced
- ½ c. chicken broth
- ½ lb. or 220 g cooked chicken
- 1 tbsp. olive oil
- 4 oz. or 113g shrimp
- Salt and black pepper
- 1 diced sweet potato
- 2 eggs
- ¼ tsp. cayenne pepper
- 2 tsps. garlic powder
- 1 c. fresh spinach

Directions:

1. In a skillet, add the olive oil. Fry the shrimp, cooked chicken and sweet potato for 2 minutes. Add the cayenne pepper, garlic powder and toss for 4 minutes. Add the zucchini and toss for another 3 minutes.
2. Whisk the eggs in a bowl and add to the skillet. Season using salt and pepper. Cover with the lid. Cook for 1 more minute and mix in the chicken broth.

3. Cover and cook for another 8 minutes on high heat. Add the spinach, toss for 2 more minutes and serve.

Nutrition (for 100g):

198 Calories

0.7g Fat

7g Carbohydrates

10g Protein

725mg Sodium

54. Basil and Tomato Soup

Preparation Time: 10 minutes

Cooking Time: 25 minutes

Servings: 2

Ingredients

- 2 tbsps. vegetable broth
- 1 minced garlic clove
- ½ c. white onion
- 1 chopped celery stalk
- 1 chopped carrot
- 3 c. tomatoes, chopped
- Salt and pepper
- 2 bay leaves
- 1 ½ c. unsweetened almond milk
- 1/3 c. basil leaves

Directions:

1. Cook the vegetable broth in a large saucepan over medium heat. Add in garlic and onions and cook for 4 minutes. Add in carrots and celery. Cook for 1 more minute.
2. Put in the tomatoes and bring to a boil. Simmer for 15 minutes. Add the almond milk, basil and bay leaves. Season it and serve.

Nutrition (for 100g):

213 Calories

3.9g Fat

9g Carbohydrates

11g Protein

817mg Sodium

55. Butternut Squash Hummus

Preparation Time: 10 minutes

Cooking Time: 15 minutes

Servings: 4

Ingredients

- 2 lbs. or 900 g seeded butternut squash, peeled
- 1 tbsp. olive oil
- ¼ c. tahini
- 2 tbsps. lemon juice
- 2 minced cloves garlic
- Salt and pepper

Directions:

1. Heat the oven to 300 F/148 C. Coat the butternut squash with olive oil. Set in a baking dish to bake for 15 minutes in the oven. When the squash is cooked, incorporate in a food processor together with the rest of the ingredients.
2. Pulse until smooth. Serve with carrots and celery sticks. For further use of place in individual containers, put a label and store it in the fridge. Allow warming at room temperature before heating in the microwave oven.

Nutrition (for 100g):

115 Calories

5.8g Fat

6.7g Carbohydrates

10g Protein

946mg Sodium

56. Ham Muffins

Preparation Time: 10 minutes

Cooking Time: 15 minutes

Servings: 6

Ingredients

- 9 ham slices
- 1/3 c. chopped spinach
- ¼ c. crumbled feta cheese
- ½ c. chopped roasted red peppers
- Salt and black pepper
- 1½ tbsps. basil pesto
- 5 whisked eggs

Directions:

1. Grease a muffin tin. Use 1 ½ ham slices to line each of the muffin molds. Except for black pepper, salt, pesto, and eggs, divide the rest of the ingredients into your ham cups. Using a bowl, whisk together the pepper, salt, pesto, and eggs. Pour your pepper mixture on top. Set oven to 400 F/204 C and bake for about 15 minutes. Serve immediately.

Nutrition (for 100g):

109 Calories

6.7g Fat

1.8g Carbohydrates

9g Protein

386mg Sodium

57. Farro Salad

Preparation Time: 10 minutes

Cooking Time: 0 minute

Servings: 2

Ingredients

- 1 tbsp. olive oil
- Salt and black pepper
- 1 bunch baby spinach, chopped
- 1 pitted avocado, peeled and chopped
- 1 minced garlic clove
- 2 c. cooked farro
- ½ c. cherry tomatoes, cubed

Directions:

2. Adjust your heat to medium. Set oil in a pan and heat. Toss in the rest of the ingredients. Cook the mixture for approximately 5 minutes. Set in serving plates and enjoy.

Nutrition (for 100g):

157 Calories

13.7g Fat

5.5g Carbohydrates

6g Protein

615mg Sodium

58. Cranberry and Dates Squares

Preparation Time: 10 minutes

Cooking Time: 20 minutes

Servings: 10

Ingredients

- 12 pitted dates, chopped
- 1 tsp. vanilla extract
- ¼ c. honey
- ½ c. rolled oats
- ¾ c. dried cranberries
- ¼ c. melted almond avocado oil
- 1 c. chopped walnuts, roasted
- ¼ c. pumpkin seeds

Directions:

1. Using a bowl, stir in all ingredients to mix.
2. Line a parchment paper on a baking sheet. Press the mixture on the setup. Set in your freezer for about 30 minutes. Slice into 10 squares and enjoy.

Nutrition (for 100g):

263 Calories

13.4g Fat

14.3g Carbohydrates

7g Protein

845mg Sodium

59. Lentils and Cheddar Frittata

Preparation Time: 5 minutes

Cooking Time: 17 minutes

Servings: 4

Ingredients

- 1 chopped red onion
- 2 tbsps. olive oil
- 1 c. boiled sweet potatoes, chopped
- ¾ c. chopped ham
- 4 whisked eggs
- ¾ c. cooked lentils
- 2 tbsps. Greek yogurt
- Salt and black pepper
- ½ c. halved cherry tomatoes,
- ¾ c. grated cheddar cheese

Directions:

1. Adjust your heat to medium and set a pan in place. Add in oil to heat. Stir in onion and allow to sauté for about 2 minutes. Except for cheese and eggs, toss in the other ingredients and cook for 3 more minutes. Add in the eggs, top with cheese. Cook for 10 more minutes while covered.
2. Slice the frittata, set in serving bowls and enjoy.

Nutrition (for 100g):

274 Calories

17.3g Fat

3.5g Carbohydrates

6g Protein

843mg Sodium

60. Tuna Sandwich

Preparation Time: 5 minutes

Cooking Time: 5 minutes

Servings: 2

Ingredients

- 6 oz. or 170 g canned tuna, drained and flaked
- 1 pitted avocado, peeled and mashed
- 4 whole-wheat bread slices
- Pinch salt and black pepper
- 1 tbsp. crumbled feta cheese
- 1 c. baby spinach

Directions:

1. Using a bowl, stir in pepper, salt, tuna, and cheese to mix. To the bread slices, apply a spread of the mashed avocado.
2. Equally, divide the tuna mixture and spinach onto 2 of the slices. Top with the remaining 2 slices. Serve.

Nutrition (for 100g):

283 Calories

11.2g Fat

3.4g Carbohydrates

8g Protein

754mg Sodium

Dessert

61. Butter Pie

Preparation Time: 10 minutes

Cooking Time: 15 minutes

Servings: 2

Ingredients:

- 3 whole eggs
- 6 tbsp of all-purpose flour
- 1 ½ cup of milk
- Salt to taste
- 4 tbsp of butter
- 1 cup of skim sour cream
- 1 tbsp of ground red pepper

Directions:

1. Preheat the oven to 300°. Line in some baking paper over a baking dish and then set it aside.
2. Mix well three eggs, all-purpose flour, 2 table spoons of butter, milk, and salt. Spread the mixture on a baking dish and then bake it for about 15 minutes.
3. When done, remove from the oven and cool for a while. Chop into bite-sized pieces and place on a serving plate. Pour 1 cup of sour cream.
4. Melt the remaining 2 table spoons of butter over a medium temperature. Add 1 tablespoon of ground red pepper and stir-fry for several minutes. Drizzle some of this mixture over the pie and serve immediately.

Nutrition:

Calories 317

Fat 17g

Carbs 36g

Protein 24g

62. Homemade Spinach Pie

Preparation Time: 20 minutes

Cooking Time: 30 minutes

Servings: 5

Ingredients:

- o   lb. fresh spinach
- 0.5 lb. fresh dandelion leaves
- ¼ cup of Feta cheese, crumbled
- ½ cup of sour cream
- ½ cup of blue cheese, chopped
- 2 eggs
- 2 tbsp of butter, melted
- Salt to taste
- 1 pack of pie crust
- Vegetable oil

Directions:

2. Preheat the oven to 350 degrees. Use 1 table spoon of butter to grease the baking dish.
3. Add the ingredients in a large bowl and then mix well. Grease the pie crust with some oil. Spread the spinach mixture over the pie crust and roll. Place in a baking dish and then bake for about 30-40 minutes
4. Remove from the heat and serve warm.

Nutrition:

Calories 230

Fat 9g

Carbs 29g

Protein 11g

63. Rhubarb Strawberry Crunch

Preparation Time: 20 minutes

Cooking Time: 60 minutes

Servings: 18

Ingredients:

- 3 tbsps. all-purpose flour
- 3 c. fresh strawberries, sliced
- 3 c. rhubarb, cubed
- 1 ½ c. flour
- 1 c. packed brown sugar

- 1 c. butter
- 1 c. oatmeal

Directions:

1. Preheat the oven to 374°F
2. In a medium bowl mix rhubarb, 3 tbsps. flour, white sugar, and strawberries. Set the mixture in a baking dish.
3. In another bowl mix 1 ½ cups of flour, brown sugar, butter, and oats until a crumbly texture is obtained. You may use a blender.
4. Combine mixtures and place on the baking pan
5. Bake for 45 minutes or until crispy and light brown.

Nutrition:

Calories 253

Fat 10.8g

Carbs 38.1g

Protein 2.3g

64. Banana Dessert with Chocolate Chips

Preparation Time: 20 minutes

Cooking Time: 30 minutes

Servings: 24

Ingredients:

- 2/3 c. white sugar
- ¾ c. butter
- 2/3 c. brown sugar
- 1 egg, beaten
- 1 tsp. vanilla extract
- 1 c. banana puree
- 1 ¾ c. flour
- 2 tsps. baking powder
- ½ tsp. salt
- 1 c. semi-sweet chocolate chips

Directions:

1. Preheat oven at 350°F
2. In a bowl, add the sugars and butter and beat until lightly colored
3. Add the egg and vanilla.

4. Add the banana puree and stir
5. In another bowl mix baking powder, flour, and salt. Add this mixture to the butter mixture
6. Stir in the chocolate chips
7. Prepare a baking pan and place the dough onto it
8. Bake for 20 minutes and let it cool for 5 minutes before slicing into equal squares

Nutrition:

Calories 174

Fat 8.2g

Carbs 25.2g

Protein 1.7g

65. Cranberry and Pistachio Biscotti

Preparation Time: 20 minutes

Cooking Time: 60 minutes

Servings: 4

Ingredients:

- ¼ c. light olive oil
- ¾ c. white sugar
- 2 tsps. vanilla extract
- ½ tsp. almond extract
- 2 eggs
- 1 ¾ c. all-purpose flour
- ¼ tsp. salt
- 1 tsp. baking powder
- ½ c. dried cranberries
- 1 ½ c. pistachio nuts

Directions:

1. Preheat the oven at 300 F/ 148 C
2. Combine olive oil and sugar in a bowl and mix well
3. Add eggs, almond and vanilla extracts, stir
4. Add baking powder, salt, and flour
5. Add cranberries and nuts, mix
6. Divide the dough in half — form two 12 x 2-inch logs on a parchment baking sheet.
7. Set in the oven and bake for 35 minutes or until the blocks are golden brown. Set

from oven and allow to cool for about 10 minutes.

8. Set the oven to 275 F/ 135 C
9. Cut diagonal trunks into 3/4-inch-thick slices. Place on the sides on the baking sheet covered with parchment
10. Bake for about 8 - 10 minutes or until dry
11. You can serve it both hot and cold

Nutrition:

Calories 92

Fat 4.3g

Carbs 11.7g

Protein 2.1g

66. Mascarpone and Fig Crostini

Preparation Time: 10 minutes

Cooking Time: 10 minutes

Servings: 6-8

Ingredients:

- 1 long French baguette
- 4 tablespoons (½ stick) salted butter, melted
- 1 (8-ounce) tub mascarpone cheese
- 1 (12-ounce) jar fig jam or preserves

Directions:

1. Preheat the oven to 350°F.
2. Slice the bread into ¼-inch-thick slices.
3. Lay out the sliced bread on a single baking sheet and brush each slice with the melted butter.
4. Put the single baking sheet in the oven and toast the bread for 5 to 7 minutes, just until golden brown.
5. Let the bread cool slightly. Spread it about a tea spoon or so of the mascarpone cheese on each piece of bread.
6. Top with a teaspoon or so of the jam. Serve immediately.

Nutrition:

Calories 445

Fat 24g

Carbs 48g

Protein 3g

67. Crunchy Sesame Cookies

Preparation Time: 10 minutes

Cooking Time: 15 minutes

Servings: 14-16

Ingredients:

- 1 cup sesame seeds, hulled
- 1 cup sugar
- 8 tablespoons (1 stick) salted butter, softened
- 2 large eggs
- 1¼ cups flour

Directions:

1. Preheat the oven to 350°F. Toast the sesame seeds on a baking sheet for 3 minutes. Set aside and let cool.
2. Using a mixer, cream together the sugar and butter.
3. Put the eggs one at a time until well-blended.
4. Add the flour and toasted sesame seeds and mix until well-blended.
5. Drop spoonful of cookie dough onto a baking sheet and form them into round balls, about 1-inch in diameter, similar to a walnut.
6. Put in the oven and bake for 5 to 7 minutes or until golden brown.
7. Let the cookies cool and enjoy.

Nutrition:

Calories 218

Fat 12g

Carbs 25g

Protein 4g

68. Almond Cookies

Preparation Time: 5 minutes

Cooking Time: 10 minutes

Servings: 4-6

Ingredients:

- ½ cup sugar
- 8 tablespoons (1 stick) room temperature salted butter
- 1 large egg
- 1½ cups all-purpose flour
- 1 cup ground almonds or almond flour

Directions:

1. Preheat the oven to 375°F.
2. Using a mixer, cream together the sugar and butter.
3. Add the egg and mix until combined.
4. Alternately add the flour and ground almonds, ½ cup at a time, while the mixer is on slow.
5. Once everything is combined, line a baking sheet with parchment paper. Drop a tablespoon of dough on the baking sheet, keeping the cookies at least 2 inches apart.
6. Put the single baking sheet in the oven and bake just until the cookies start to turn brown around the edges for about 5 to 7 minutes.

Nutrition:

Calories 604

Fat 36g

Carbs 63g

Protein 11g

69. Baklava and Honey

Preparation Time: 40 minutes

Cooking Time: 1 hour

Servings: 6-8

Ingredients:

- 2 cups chopped walnuts or pecans
- 1 teaspoon cinnamon
- 1 cup of melted unsalted butter

- 1 (16-ounce) package phyllo dough, thawed
- 1 (12-ounce) jar honey

Directions:

1. Preheat the oven to 350°F.
2. In a bowl, combine the chopped nuts and cinnamon.
3. Using a brush, butter the sides and bottom of a 9-by-13-inch inch baking dish.
4. Take off the phyllo dough from the package and cut it to the size of the baking dish using a sharp knife.
5. Put one sheet of phyllo dough on the bottom of the dish, brush with butter, and repeat until you have 8 layers.
6. Sprinkle ⅓ cup of the nut mixture over the phyllo layers. Top with a sheet of phyllo dough, butter that sheet, and repeat until you have 4 sheets of buttered phyllo dough.
7. Sprinkle ⅓ cup of the nut mixture for another layer of nuts. Repeat the layering of nuts and 4 sheets of buttered phyllo until all the nut mixture is gone. The last layer should be 8 buttered sheets of phyllo.
8. Before you bake, cut the baklava into desired shapes; traditionally this is diamonds, triangles, or squares.
9. Bake the baklava for about 1 hour just until the top layer is golden brown.
10. While the baklava is baking, heat the honey in a pan just until it is warm and easy to pour.
11. Once the baklava is done baking, directly pour the honey evenly over the baklava and let it absorb it, about 20 minutes. Serve warm or at room temperature.

Nutrition:

Calories 1235

Fat 89g

Carbs 109g

Protein 18g

70. Date and Nut Balls

Preparation Time: 10 minutes

Cooking Time: 10 minutes

Servings: 6-8

Ingredients:

- 1 cup walnuts or pistachios
- 1 cup unsweetened shredded coconut
- 14 medjool dates, pits removed
- 8 tablespoons (1 stick) butter, melted

Directions:

1. Preheat the oven to 350°F.
2. Put the nuts on a baking sheet. Toast the nuts for 5 minutes.
3. Put the shredded coconut on a clean baking sheet; toast just until it turns golden brown, about 3 to 5 minutes (coconut burns fast so keep an eye on it). Once done, remove it from the oven and put it in a shallow bowl.
4. Inside a food processor with a chopping blade, put the nuts until they have a medium chop. Put the chopped nuts into a medium bowl.
5. Add the dates and melted butter to the food processor and blend until the dates become a thick paste. Pour the chopped nuts into the food processor with the dates and pulse just until the mixture is combined, about 5 to 7 pulses.
6. Remove the mixture from the food processor and scrape it into a large bowl.
7. To make the balls, spoon 1 to 2 tablespoons of the date mixture into the palm of your hand and roll around between your hands until you form a ball. Put the ball on a clean, lined baking sheet. Repeat this until all of the mixture is formed into balls.
8. Roll each ball in the toasted coconut until the outside of the ball is coated, put the ball back on the baking sheet, and repeat.
9. Put all the balls into the fridge for 20 minutes before serving so that they firm up. You can also store any leftovers inside the fridge in an airtight container.

Nutrition:

Calories 489

Fat 35g

Carbs 48g

Protein 5g

71. Creamy Rice Pudding

Preparation Time: 5 minutes

Cooking Time: 45 minutes

Servings: 6

Ingredients:

- 1¼ cups long-grain rice
- 5 cups whole milk
- 1 cup sugar
- 1 tablespoon of rose water/orange blossom water
- 1 teaspoon cinnamon

Directions:

1. Rinse the rice under cold water for 30 seconds.
2. Add the rice, milk, and sugar in a large pot. Bring to a gentle boil while continually stirring.
3. Lessen the heat to low and then let simmer for 40 to 45 minutes, stirring every 3 to 4 minutes so that the rice does not stick to the bottom of the pot.
4. Add the rose water at the end and simmer for 5 minutes.
5. Divide the pudding into 6 bowls. Sprinkle the top with cinnamon. Let it cool for over an hour before serving. Store in the fridge.

Nutrition:

Calories 394

Fat 7g

Carbs 75g

Protein 9g

72. Ricotta-Lemon Cheesecake

Preparation Time: 5 minutes

Cooking Time: 1 hour

Servings: 8-10

Ingredients:

- 2 (8-ounce) packages full-fat cream cheese
- 1 (16-ounce) container full-fat ricotta cheese
- 1½ cups granulated sugar
- 1 tablespoon lemon zest
- 5 large eggs
- Nonstick cooking spray

Directions:

1. Preheat the oven to 350°F.
2. Blend together the cream cheese and ricotta cheese.
3. Blend in the sugar and lemon zest.
4. Blend in the eggs; drop in 1 egg at a time, blend for 10 seconds, and repeat.
5. Put a 9-inch springform pan with a parchment paper and nonstick spray. Wrap the bottom of the pan with foil. Pour the cheesecake batter into the pan.
6. To make a water bath, get a baking or roasting pan larger than the cheesecake pan. Fill the roasting pan about ⅓ of the way up with warm water. Put the cheesecake pan into the water bath. Put the whole thing in the oven and let the cheesecake bake for 1 hour.
7. After baking is complete, remove the cheesecake pan from the water bath and remove the foil. Let the cheese cake cool for 1 hour on the countertop. Then put it in the fridge to cool for at least 3 hours before serving.

Nutrition:

Calories 489

Fat 31g

Carbs 42g

Protein 15g

73. Crockpot Keto Chocolate Cake

Preparation Time: 20 minutes

Cooking Time: 3 hours

Servings: 12

Ingredients:

- ¾ c. stevia sweetener
- 1 ½ c. almond flour
- ¼ tsp. baking powder
- ¼ c. protein powder, chocolate, or vanilla flavor
- 2/3 c. unsweetened cocoa powder
- ¼ tsp. salt
- ½ c. unsalted butter, melted
- 4 large eggs
- ¾ c. heavy cream
- 1 tsp. vanilla extract

Directions:

1. Grease the ceramic insert of the Crockpot.
2. In a bowl, mix the sweetener, almond flour, protein powder, cocoa powder, salt, and baking powder.
3. Add the butter, eggs, cream, and vanilla extract.
4. Pour the batter in the Crockpot and cook on low for 3 hours.
5. Allow to cool before slicing.

Nutrition:

Calories: 253

Carbohydrates: 5.1g

Protein: 17.3g

Fat: 29.5g

74. Keto Crockpot Chocolate Lava Cake

Preparation Time: 30 minutes

Cooking Time: 3 hours

Servings: 12

Ingredients:

- 1 ½ c. stevia sweetener, divided
- ½ c. almond flour
- 5 tbsps. unsweetened cocoa powder
- ½ tsp. salt
- 1 tsp. baking powder
- 3 whole eggs
- 3 egg yolks
- ½ c. butter, melted
- 1 tsp. vanilla extract
- 2 c. hot water
- 4 ounces sugar-free chocolate chips

Directions:

1. Grease the inside of the Crockpot.
2. In a bowl, mix the stevia sweetener, almond flour, cocoa powder, salt, and baking powder.
3. In another bowl, mix the eggs, egg yolks, butter, and vanilla extract. Pour in the hot water.
4. Pour the wet ingredients to the dry ingredients and fold to create a batter.
5. Add the chocolate chips last
6. Pour into the greased Crockpot and cook on low for 3 hours.
7. Allow to cool before serving.

Nutrition:

Calories: 157

Carbohydrates: 5.5g

Protein: 10.6g

Fat: 13g

75. Lemon Crockpot Cake

Preparation Time: 15 minutes

Cooking Time: 3 hours

Servings: 8

Ingredients:

- ½ c. coconut flour
- 1 ½ c. almond flour
- 3 tbsps. stevia sweetener
- 2 tsps. baking powder
- ½ tsp. xanthan gum
- ½ c. whipping cream
- ½ c. butter, melted
- 1 tbsp. juice, freshly squeezed
- Zest from one large lemon
- 2 eggs

Directions:

1. Grease the inside of the Crockpot with a butter or cooking spray.
2. Mix together coconut flour, almond flour, stevia, baking powder, and xanthan gum in a bowl.
3. In another bowl, combine the whipping cream, butter, lemon juice, lemon zest, and eggs. Mix until well combined.
4. Pour the wet ingredients to the dry ingredients gradually and fold to create a smooth batter.
5. Spread the batter in the Crockpot and cook on low for 3 hours

Nutrition:

Calories: 350

Carbohydrates: 11.1g

Protein: 17.6g

Fat: 32.6g

76. Lemon and Watermelon Granita

Preparation Time: 10 minutes + 3 hours to freeze

Cooking Time: None

Servings: 4

Ingredients:

- 4 cups watermelon cubes
- ¼ cup honey
- ¼ cup freshly squeezed lemon juice

Directions:

1. In a blender, combine the watermelon, honey, and lemon juice. Purée all the ingredients, then pour into a 9-by-9-by-2-inch baking pan and place in the freezer.

2. Every 30 to 60 minutes, run a fork across the frozen surface to fluff and create ice flakes. Freeze for about 3 hours total and serve.

Nutrition:

Calories: 153

Carbohydrates: 39g

Protein: 2g

Fat: 1g

77. Baked Apples with Walnuts and Spices

Preparation Time: 10 minutes

Cooking Time: 45 minutes

Servings: 4

Ingredients:

- 4 apples
- ¼ cup chopped walnuts
- 2 tablespoons honey
- 1 teaspoon ground cinnamon
- ¼ teaspoon ground nutmeg
- ¼ teaspoon ground ginger
- Pinch sea salt

Directions:

1. Preheat the oven to 375°F.
2. Cut the tops off the apples and then use a metal spoon or a paring knife to remove the cores, leaving the bottoms of the apples intact. Place the apples cut-side up in a 9-by-9-inch baking pan.
3. Stir together the walnuts, honey, cinnamon, nutmeg, ginger, and sea salt. Put the mixture into the centers of the apples. Bake the apples for about 45 minutes until browned, soft, and fragrant. Serve warm.

Nutrition:

Calories: 199

Carbohydrates: 41g

Protein: 5g

Fat: 5g

78. Red Wine Poached Pears

Preparation Time: 10 minutes

Cooking Time: 45 minutes + 3 hours to chill

Servings: 4

Ingredients:

- 2 cups dry red wine
- ¼ cup honey
- Zest of ½ orange
- 2 cinnamon sticks
- 1 (1-inch) piece fresh ginger
- 4 pears, bottom inch sliced off so the pear is flat

Directions:

1. In a pot on medium-high heat, stir together the wine, honey, orange zest, cinnamon, and ginger. Bring to a boil, stirring occasionally. Lessen the heat to medium-low and then simmer for 5 minutes to let the flavors blend.
2. Add the pears to the pot. Cover and simmer for 20 minutes until the pears are tender, turning every 3 to 4 minutes to ensure even color and contact with the liquid. Refrigerate the pears in the liquid for 3 hours to allow for more flavor absorption.
3. Bring the pears and liquid to room temperature. Place the pears on individual dishes and return the poaching liquid to the stove top over medium-high heat. Simmer for 15 minutes until the liquid is syrupy. Serve the pears with the liquid drizzled over the top.

Nutrition:

Calories: 283

Carbohydrates: 53g

Protein: 1g

Fat: 1g

79. Vanilla Pudding with Strawberries

Preparation Time: 10 minutes

Cooking Time: 10 minutes + chilling time

Servings: 4

Ingredients:

2¼ cups skim milk, divided

1 egg, beaten

½ cup sugar

1 teaspoon vanilla extract

Pinch sea salt

3 tablespoons cornstarch

2 cups sliced strawberries

Directions:

1. In a small bowl, whisk 2 cups of milk with the egg, sugar, vanilla, and sea salt. Transfer the mixture to a medium pot, place it over medium heat, and slowly bring to a boil, whisking constantly.
2. Whisk the cornstarch with the ¼ cup of milk. In a thin stream, whisk this slurry into the boiling mixture in the pot. Cook until it thickens, stirring constantly. Boil for 1 minute more, stirring constantly.
3. Spoon the pudding into 4 dishes and refrigerate to chill. Serve topped with the sliced strawberries.

Nutrition:

Calories: 209

Carbohydrates: 43g

Protein: 6g

Fat: 1g

80. Mixed Berry Frozen Yogurt Bar

Preparation Time: 10 minutes

Cooking Time: None

Servings: 8

Ingredients:

- 8 cups low-fat vanilla frozen yogurt (or flavor of choice)
- 1 cup sliced fresh strawberries
- 1 cup fresh blueberries
- 1 cup fresh blackberries
- 1 cup fresh raspberries
- ½ cup chopped walnuts

Directions:

1. Apportion the yogurt among 8 dessert bowls. Serve the toppings family style, and let your guests choose their toppings and spoon them over the yogurt.

Nutrition:

Calories: 81

Carbohydrates: 9g

Protein: 3g

Fat: 5g

81. Fruit Salad with Yogurt Cream

Preparation Time: 10 minutes

Cooking Time: None

Servings: 4

Ingredients:

- 1½ cups grapes, halved
- 1 cup chopped cantaloupe
- 2 plums, chopped
- 1 peach, chopped
- ½ cup fresh blueberries
- 1 cup unsweetened plain nonfat Greek yogurt
- 2 tablespoons honey
- ½ teaspoon ground cinnamon

Directions:

2. In a large bowl, combine the grapes, cantaloupe, plums, peach, and blueberries. Toss to mix. Divide among 4 dessert dishes.
3. Whisk the yogurt, honey, and cinnamon. Spoon over the fruit.

Nutrition:

Calories: 159

Carbohydrates: 38g

Protein: 3g

Fat: 1g

82. Date Nut Energy Balls

Preparation Time: 10 minutes

Cooking Time: None

Servings: 24

Ingredients:

- 1 cup walnuts
- 1 cup almonds
- 2 cups Medjool dates, pitted
- 2 tablespoons extra-virgin olive oil
- ¼ cup unsweetened cocoa powder
- ¼ cup shredded unsweetened coconut, plus additional for coating
- Pinch sea salt

Directions:

1. Combine the walnuts, almonds, dates, olive oil, cocoa powder, coconut, and sea salt. Pulse for 20 to 30 (1-second pulses) until everything is well chopped. Form the mixture into 24 balls.
2. Spread the additional coconut on a plate and roll the balls in the coconut to coat. Serve, refrigerate, or freeze.

Nutrition:

Calories: 164

Carbohydrates: 26g

Protein: 3g

Fat: 6g

83. Pastaflora

Preparation Time: 15 minutes

Cooking Time: 35 minutes

Servings: 24

Ingredients:

- Nonstick cooking spray
- 2 cups all-purpose flour
- ½ cup sugar
- 1 teaspoon vanilla extract
- ½ cup (1 stick) unsalted butter
- 2 teaspoons baking powder
- 2 eggs
- 2 tablespoons orange zest
- ¼ cup apricot jam

Directions:

1. Preheat the oven to 400°F.
2. Coat a 9-by-13-inch baking dish with a cooking spray.
3. Combine the flour, sugar, vanilla, butter, baking powder, eggs, and orange zest. Pulse until a stiff dough forms. Press three-fourths of the dough into the prepared dish.
4. Spread the jam over the dough.
5. Roll out the remaining dough to ¼-inch thickness and cut it into ½-inch-wide strips. Form a lattice on top of the jam with the strips. Bake for about 35 minutes until golden. Cool on a wire rack.
6. Cut into 24 cookies and serve.

Nutrition:

Calories: 102

Carbohydrates: 15g

Protein: 2g

Fat: 4g

84. Blueberry-Blackberry Ice Pops

Preparation Time: 5 minutes + 2 hours to freeze

Cooking Time: None

Servings: 2

Ingredients:

- ½ (13.5-ounce) can coconut cream, ¾ cup unsweetened full-fat coconut milk, or ¾ cup heavy (whipping) cream

- 2 teaspoons Swerve natural sweetener or 2 drops liquid stevia
- ½ teaspoon vanilla extract
- ¼ cup mixed blueberries and blackberries

Directions:

1. Add together the coconut cream, sweetener, and vanilla.
2. Add the mixed berries, and then pulse just a few times.
3. Pour it into ice pop molds and freeze for at least about 2 hours before serving.

Nutrition:

Calories: 165

Carbohydrates: 4g

Protein: 1g

Fat: 17g

85. Strawberry-Lime Ice Pops

Preparation Time: 5 minutes + 2 hours to freeze

Cooking Time: None

Servings: 4

Ingredients:

- ½ (13.5-ounce) can coconut cream, ¾ cup unsweetened full-fat coconut milk, or ¾ cup heavy (whipping) cream
- 2 teaspoons Swerve natural sweetener or 2 drops liquid stevia
- 1 tablespoon freshly squeezed lime juice
- ¼ cup hulled and sliced strawberries (fresh or frozen)

Directions:

1. Mix together the coconut cream, sweetener, and lime juice in a blend
2. Add the strawberries, and pulse just a few times so the strawberries retain their texture.
3. Pour into ice pop molds, and freeze for at least 2 hours before serving.

Nutrition:

Calories: 166

Carbohydrates: 5g

Protein: 1g

Fat: 17g

86. Coffee Ice Pops

Preparation Time: 5 minutes + 2 hours to freeze

Cooking Time: None

Servings: 4

Ingredients:

- 2 cups brewed coffee, cold
- ¾ cup coconut cream, ¾ cup unsweetened full-fat coconut milk, or ¾ cup heavy (whipping) cream
- 2 teaspoons Swerve natural sweetener or 2 drops liquid stevia
- 2 tablespoons sugar-free chocolate chips (I use Lily's)

Directions:

1. Mix together the coffee, coconut cream, and sweetener until thoroughly blended.
2. Flow it into ice pop molds, and then drop a few chocolate chips into each mold.
3. Freeze for at least about 2 hours before serving.

Nutrition:

Calories: 105

Carbohydrates: 7g

Protein: 1g

Fat: 10g

87. Fudge Ice Pops

Preparation Time: 5 minutes + 2 hours to freeze

Cooking Time: None

Servings: 4

Ingredients:

½ (13.5-ounce) can coconut cream, ¾ cup unsweetened full-fat coconut milk, or ¾ cup heavy (whipping) cream

2 teaspoons Swerve natural sweetener or 2 drops liquid stevia

2 tablespoons unsweetened cocoa powder

2 tablespoons sugar-free chocolate chips (I use Lily's)

Directions:

1. Mix together the coconut cream, sweetener, and unsweetened cocoa powder.
2. Pour into ice pop molds, and drop chocolate chips into each mold.
3. Let it freeze for at least about 2 hours before serving.

Nutrition:

Calories: 193

Carbohydrates: 9g

Protein: 2g

Fat: 20g

88. Root Beer Float

Preparation Time: 5 minutes

Cooking Time: 30 minutes

Servings: 2

Ingredients:

- 1 (12-ounce) can diet root beer (I like Zevia's)
- 4 tablespoons heavy (whipping) cream
- 1 teaspoon vanilla extract
- 6 ice cubes

Directions:

1. Combine the root beer, cream, vanilla, and ice.
2. Blend it well, pour into two tall glasses, and then serve.
3. For me, no root beer float is complete without a bendy straw.

Nutrition:

Calories: 56

Carbohydrates: 3g

Protein: 1g

Fat: 6g

89. Orange Cream Float

Preparation Time: 5 minutes

Cooking Time: 30 minutes

Servings: 2

Ingredients:

- 1 can diet orange soda (I like Zevia's)
- 4 tablespoons heavy (whipping) cream
- 1 teaspoon vanilla extract
- 6 ice cubes

Directions:

1. Combine the orange soda, cream, vanilla, and ice.
2. Blend it well, pour into two tall glasses, and then serve.

Nutrition:

Calories: 56

Carbohydrates: 3g

Protein: 1g

Fat: 6g

90. Strawberry Shake

Preparation Time: 10 minutes

Cooking Time: 30 minutes

Servings: 2

Ingredients:

- ¾ cup heavy (whipping) cream
- 2 ounces cream cheese, at room temperature
- 1 tablespoon Swerve natural sweetener
- ¼ teaspoon vanilla extract

- 6 strawberries, sliced
- 6 ice cubes

Directions:

1. Combine the heavy cream, cream cheese, sweetener, and vanilla. Mix on high to fully combine.
2. Add the strawberries and ice, and then blend until smooth.
3. Pour into two tall glasses and serve.

Nutrition:

Calories: 407

Carbohydrates: 13g

Protein: 4g

Fat: 42g

91. "Frosty" Chocolate Shake

Preparation Time: 10 minutes + 1 hour to chill

Cooking Time: None

Servings: 2

Ingredients:

- ¾ cup heavy (whipping) cream
- 4 ounces coconut milk
- 1 tablespoon Swerve natural sweetener
- ¼ teaspoon vanilla extract
- 2 tablespoons unsweetened cocoa powder

Directions:

1. Pour the cream into a medium cold metal bowl, and with your hand mixer and cold beaters, beat the cream just until it forms peaks.
2. Slowly pour in the coconut milk, and gently stir it into the cream. Add the sweetener, vanilla, and cocoa powder, and beat until fully combined.
3. Pour into two tall glasses, and chill in the freezer for 1 hour before serving. I usually stir the shakes twice during this time.

Nutrition:

Calories: 444

Carbohydrates: 15g

Protein: 4g

Fat: 47g

92. Strawberry Cheesecake Mousse

Preparation Time: 10 minutes + 1 hour to chill

Cooking Time: None

Servings: 2

Ingredients:

- 4 ounces cream cheese, at room temperature
- 1 tablespoon heavy (whipping) cream
- 1 teaspoon Swerve natural sweetener or 1 drop liquid stevia
- 1 teaspoon vanilla extract
- 4 strawberries, sliced (fresh or frozen)

Directions:

1. Chop the cream cheese block into smaller pieces and distribute evenly in a food processor (or blender). Add the cream, sweetener, and vanilla.
2. Mix together on high. I usually stop and stir twice and scrape down the sides of the bowl with a small rubber scraper to make it sure everything is mixed very well.
3. Add the strawberries into the food processor, and then mix until combined.
4. Divide the strawberry cheesecake mixture between two small dishes, and then chill for a 1 hour before serving.

Nutrition:

Calories: 221

Carbohydrates: 11g

Protein: 4g

Fat: 21g

93. Lemonade Fat Bomb

Preparation Time: 10 minutes + 2 hour to freeze

Cooking Time: None

Servings: 2

Ingredients:

- ½ lemon
- 4 ounces cream cheese, at room temperature
- 2 ounces butter, at room temperature
- 2 teaspoons Swerve natural sweetener or 2 drops liquid stevia
- Pinch pink Himalayan salt

Directions:

1. Zest the lemon half with a very fine grater into a small bowl. Squeeze the juice of the lemon in the bowl with the zest.
2. In a medium bowl, combine the cream cheese and butter. Add the sweetener, lemon zest and juice, and pink Himalayan salt. Using a hand mixer, beat until fully combined.
3. Spoon the mixture into the fat bomb molds. (I use small silicone cupcake molds. If you don't have molds, you can use cupcake paper liners that fit into the cups of a muffin tin.)
4. Freeze for at least about 2 hours and eat! Keep extras in your freezer in a zip-top bag so you and your loved ones can have them anytime you are craving a sweet treat. They will keep in the freezer for up to 3 months.

Nutrition:

Calories: 404

Carbohydrates: 8g

Protein: 4g

Fat: 43g

94. Berry Cheesecake Fat Bomb

Preparation Time: 10 minutes + 2 hour to freeze

Cooking Time: None

Servings: 2

Ingredients:

- 4 ounces cream cheese, at room temperature
- 4 tablespoons (½ stick) butter, at room temperature
- 2 teaspoons Swerve natural sweetener or 2 drops liquid stevia
- 1 teaspoon vanilla extract
- ¼ cup berries, fresh or frozen

Directions:

1. Apply a hand mixer to beat the cream cheese, butter, sweetener, and vanilla.
2. In a bowl, mash the berries. Put the berries into the cream-cheese mixture using a rubber scraper. (If you put slices of berries in the cream-cheese mixture without mashing them, they will freeze and have an off-putting texture.)
3. Put the cream-cheese mixture into fat bomb molds. (I use small silicone cupcake molds, which I put in the cups of a muffin tin. You can just use cupcake papers if you don't have molds.)
4. Let it freeze for at least about 2 hours, unmold them, and then eat! Leftover fat bombs can be stored in the freezer in a zip-top bag for up to 3 months.

Nutrition:

Calories: 414

Carbohydrates: 9g

Protein: 4g

Fat: 43g

95. Peanut Butter Fat Bomb

Preparation Time: 10 minutes + 30 minutes to freeze

Cooking Time: None

Servings: 2

Ingredients:

- 1 tablespoon butter, at room temperature
- 1 tablespoon coconut oil

- 2 tablespoons of all-natural peanut butter/almond butter
- 2 teaspoons Swerve natural sweetener or 2 drops liquid stevia

Directions:

1. In a microwave-safe medium bowl, melt the butter, coconut oil, and peanut butter in the microwave on 50 percent power. Mix in the sweetener.
2. Pour the mixture into fat bomb molds. (I use small silicone cupcake molds.)
3. Freeze for 30 minutes, unmold them, and eat! Keep some extras in your freezer so you can eat them anytime you are craving a sweet treat.

Nutrition:

Calories: 196

Carbohydrates: 8g

Protein: 3g

Fat: 20g

96. Crustless Cheesecake Bites

Preparation Time: 10 minutes + 3 hours to chill

Cooking Time: 30 minutes

Servings: 4

Ingredients:

- 4 ounces cream cheese, at room temperature
- ¼ cup sour cream
- 2 large eggs
- ⅓ cup Swerve natural sweetener
- ¼ teaspoon vanilla extract

Directions:

1. Preheat the oven to 350°F.
2. In a bowl, app a hand mixer to beat the cream cheese, sour cream, eggs, sweetener, and vanilla until well mixed.
3. Place silicone liners (or cupcake paper liners) in the cups of a muffin tin.

4. Pour the cheesecake batter into the liners, and bake for 30 minutes.
5. Refrigerate until completely cooled before serving, about 3 hours. Store extra cheesecake bites in a zip-top bag in the freezer for up to 3 months.

Nutrition:

Calories: 169

Carbohydrates: 18g

Protein: 5g

Fat: 15g

97. Pumpkin Crustless Cheesecake Bites

Preparation Time: 10 minutes + 3 hours to chill

Cooking Time: 30 minutes

Servings: 4

Ingredients:

- 4 ounces pumpkin purée
- 4 ounces cream cheese, at room temperature
- 2 large eggs
- ⅓ cup Swerve natural sweetener
- 2 teaspoons pumpkin pie spice

Directions:

1. Preheat the oven to 350°F.
2. In a bowl, apply a hand mixer to mix the pumpkin purée, cream cheese, eggs, sweetener, and pumpkin pie spice until thoroughly combined.
3. Place silicone liners (or cupcake paper liners) into the cups of a muffin tin.
4. Put the batter into the liners, and then bake for 30 minutes.
5. Refrigerate until completely cooled before serving, about 3 hours. Put leftover cheesecake bites in a zip-top plastic bag and store in the freezer for up to 3 months.

Nutrition:

Calories: 156

Carbohydrates: 21g

Protein: 5g

Fat: 12g

98. Berry-Pecan Mascarpone Bowl

Preparation Time: 5 minutes

Cooking Time: 30 minutes

Servings: 2

Ingredients:

- 1 cup chopped pecans
- 1 teaspoon Swerve natural sweetener or 1 drop liquid stevia
- ¼ cup mascarpone
- 30 Lily's dark-chocolate chips
- 6 strawberries, sliced

Directions:

1. Divide the pecans between two dessert bowls.
2. In a small bowl, mix the sweetener into the mascarpone cheese. Top the nuts with a dollop of the sweetened mascarpone.
3. Sprinkle in the chocolate chips, top each dish with the strawberries, and serve.

Nutrition:

Calories: 462

Carbohydrates: 15g

Protein: 6g

Fat: 47g

99. Peanut Butter Cookies

Preparation Time: 5 minutes

Cooking Time: 10 minutes + 10 minutes to cool

Servings: Makes 15 cookies

Ingredients:

- 1 cup natural crunchy peanut butter
- ½ cup Swerve natural sweetener
- 1 egg

Directions:

1. Preheat the oven to 350°F. Line a single baking sheet with a silicone baking mat or parchment paper.
2. In a bowl, use a hand mixer to mix together the peanut butter, sweetener, and egg.
3. Roll up the batter into small balls about 1 inch in diameter.
4. Spread out the cookie-dough balls on the prepared pan. Press each dough ball down with the tines of a fork, then repeat to make a crisscross pattern.
5. Bake it for at least about 12 minutes or until it is golden.
6. Let the cookies cool for 10 minutes on the lined pan before serving.

Nutrition:

Calories: 98

Carbohydrates: 10g

Protein: 4g

Fat: 8g

100.   Scallops with Beurre Blanc Sauce

Preparation Time: 5 minutes

Cooking Time: 47 minutes

Servings: 2

Ingredients:

- Beurre Blanc sauce:
- ½ teaspoon olive oil
- 1 tablespoon shallots, finely chopped
- 1 tablespoon capers
- ½ cup white wine
- ½ bar of cold butter, chopped (¼ cup)
- 1 tablespoon orange juice
- Scallops and Companions:
- ¾ pound parsnip, peeled and sliced
- ½ pound brussels sprouts, stems removed and halved
- 2 cups heavy cream
- 1-pound scallops
- 1 tablespoon olive oil

- Salt and black pepper to taste

Directions:

Beurre Blanc Sauce:

1. Cut the ingredients according to the instructions. Preheat the 8-inch skillet at medium-high temperature for 2 minutes. Add ½ teaspoon olive oil, shallots and capers; Skip for 1 minute. Add the wine and reduce the temperature to medium; cook for 4 minutes, or until 2 table spoons of liquid are left in the pan.
2. Reduce the temperature to low and slowly add the cold butter, while constantly beating with a balloon whisk.
3. Once all the butter has melted, slowly add the orange juice, while stirring. Remove the pan from the stove, cover and keep the sauce hot.
4. Scallops and Companions:
5. In the pot, add the white turnip and double cream; Cover with the valve closed and cook at medium-low temperature for 20 minutes or until soft.
6. Blend the turnip cooked with salt and enough cream to acquire the consistency of creamy mashed potatoes.
7. In the same pot (previously washed), add the cabbage and 3 tablespoons of water; Cover with the valve open and cook at medium-high temperature until it whistles (approximately 6 minutes). Reduce the temperature to low and, when the valve stops whistling, close it and cook for 4 more minutes. Remove the pot from the stove and keep the cabbages warm until serving time.
8. Preheat the skillet with 1 tablespoon of olive oil at medium-high temperature for 3 minutes. Add the scallops (previously seasoned with salt and pepper to taste), reduce the temperature to medium and then cook it for 3 minutes per side or until cooked.

Nutrition:

Calories: 644

Carbohydrates: 5 g

Protein: 32 g

Fat: 55 g

101.   Mango Snow

Preparation Time: 5 minutes

Cooking Time: 2 hours

Servings: 8

Ingredients:

- 4 cups frozen mango in pieces
- 1 can of condensed milk (14 ounces/396 g)
- 1 can of evaporated milk (12 ounces /340 g)
- Mint leaves (decoration)
- Cookies (decoration)

Directions:

1. Blend the mango and the two milks at high speed for 5 minutes.
2. Transfer the mixture to the Mixing Bowl. Cover and let cool for at least 2 hours in the freezer.
3. Garnish with mint leaves and cookies.

Nutrition:

Calories: 411

Carbohydrates: 84 g

Protein: 1 g

Fat: 8 g

102.   Cassava Cake

Preparation Time: None

Cooking Time: 27 minutes

Servings: 8

Ingredients:

- 1-pound (½ kg) of lean ground beef (90% meat)
- 3 pounds (1½ kg) of cassava, peeled and chopped into medium pieces
- ½ cup diced green pepper
- ½ cup diced red pepper

- ¼ cup diced onion
- ¼ cup stuffed olives, chopped in half
- 1 teaspoon finely chopped garlic
- 1 teaspoon hot pepper, finely chopped (optional)
- ½ cup ketchup
- ¼ cup sun-dried tomatoes
- ¼ cup small capers
- 1 cup evaporated milk
- 1 cup grated Parmesan cheese
- 1 cup Grated cheddar cheese
- Salt and black pepper to taste

Directions:

1. In the pot, add the cassava pieces (already peeled) and 1 cup of water. Cover with the valve open and cook at medium-high temperature until it whistles (in about 6 minutes). Reduce the temperature to low and, when the valve stops whistling, close it and cook for 14 more minutes.
2. Meanwhile, preheat the pot at medium-high temperature for about 3 minutes, or until a few drops of water are sprayed, they bounce off the surface without evaporating. Add the meat and cook it for 3 minutes, while stirring.
3. If you wish, you can transfer it to the small strainer to drain the excess fat that it gives off with cooking. When you're done, put it back in the same pan.
4. Add the rest of the ingredients to the meat (except evaporated milk and cheese), stir well, and cover with the valve closed. Cook for 3 more minutes at low temperature. Adjust the seasoning if necessary. Transfer the meat to Mixing Bowl and set aside.
5. When the cassava is ready, drain it with the large strainer. Remove the heart from all the pieces and place them in the Mixing Bowl. Crush well with the Round Crusher with Holes. Put evaporated milk, salt and the pepper to taste. Stir to form a homogeneous and thick puree.
6. Carefully clean the same pan where you cooked the meat with a paper towel. Spread half of the cassava uniformly, until the base is covered. Distribute all ground beef on top.

7. Mix the Parmesan cheese with the Cheddar cheese, and spread half over the meat layer.
8. Make another layer with the remaining mash and cover with the cheese. Cover the pan with the valve closed and cook at a low temperature for at least about 5 to 7 minutes or when the cheese has melted. Enjoy.

Nutrition:

Calories: 257

Carbohydrates: 34 g

Protein: 12 g

Fat: 12 g

103.   Kingly Kalamata Karithopita

Preparation Time: 15 minutes

Cooking Time: 40 minutes

Servings: 16

Ingredients:

- For the Karithopita (Walnut Cake with Syrup):
- 1¼-cups whole-wheat flour
- 1-tsp ground cinnamon
- 1-tsp baking powder
- ¾-cup white sugar
- ½-tsp salt
- ¼-tsp ground cloves
- ⅓-cup extra-virgin olive oil (as shortening)
- ¾-cup milk
- 1-pc egg, whisked
- 1-cup walnuts, finely chopped
- For the Honey-Lemon Syrup:
- ¼-cup white sugar
- ¼-cup water
- 1-tsp lemon juice
- ¼-cup honey

Directions:

1. Preheat your oven to 350 °F. Prepare a greased 9" x 9" baking pan. Set aside.

2. Combine and mix the first six Karithopita ingredients in a medium-sized mixing bowl. Mix well until fully incorporated. Transfer the mixture in the mixing bowl of your stand mixer.
3. Pour in the oil, milk, and the egg. Beat the mixture on low speed for 1 minute to a creamy and thick consistency, scraping the bottom of the mixing bowl once to avoid lumps.
4. Stir in the chopped walnuts manually using a spatula. Transfer the batter in the prepared baking pan and spread evenly.
5. Place the pan in the preheated oven. Bake for at least about 40 minutes or until an inserted toothpick into the center of the walnut cake comes out clean.
6. Let the walnut cake in the pan cool for 30 minutes. In the meantime, prepare the honey lemon syrup.
7. For the Lemon Honey-Syrup:
8. Stir in the white sugar with water in a saucepan placed over medium heat. Bring the mixture to a boil. Reduce the heat to low and then allow it simmering for 5 minutes.
9. Stir in the lemon juice and honey. Remove the saucepan from the heat.
10. By using a knife, make small slashes in a diamond pattern on the top of the cake. Pour the hot syrup over the walnut cake.

Nutrition:

Calories: 198

Carbohydrates: 26.1 g

Protein: 2.9 g

Fat: 9.8 g

104. Apple Applied Cinnamon Cake Cooked with Olive Oil

Preparation Time: 20 minutes

Cooking Time: 1 hour

Servings: 12 slices

Ingredients:

- 4-eggs
- 1-cup brown sugar +2-tbsp for apples
- 1-cup extra-virgin olive oil (as shortening)
- 1-cup milk
- 2-tsp baking powder
- 2½-cups whole-wheat flour
- 1-tsp vanilla extract
- 4-pcs apples, peeled, cored, halved, and sliced thinly
- 1½-tsp ground cinnamon
- ½-cup walnuts, chopped
- ½-cup raisins
- 3-tbsp sesame seeds

Directions:

1. Preheat your oven to 375 °F. Prepare a greased 9" x 9" baking pan. Set aside.
2. By using your electric hand mixer, beat the eggs and a cup of sugar for 10 minutes. Pour in the olive oil and beat the mixture for 3 minutes.
3. Pour in the milk, and add the baking powder, wheat flour, and vanilla. Beat the mixture for another 3 minutes.
4. Transfer half of the batter in the prepared baking pan and spread evenly.
5. Combine and mix the apples, cinnamon, walnuts, raisins, and the 2-tbsp of brown sugar in a mixing bowl. Mix thoroughly until fully combined.
6. Transfer the apple mixture over the batter in the baking pan and spread evenly.
7. Top the apple mixture with the remaining batter. Sprinkle the batter with the sesame seeds.
8. Place the pan in the preheated oven. Bake it for at least about 50 minutes or when an inserted toothpick into the center of the apple-cinnamon cake comes out clean.

Nutrition:

Calories: 420

Carbohydrates: 49.6 g

Protein: 7.3 g

Fat: 23.3 g

Vegetables

105.   Portobello Caprese

Preparation Time: 15 minutes

Cooking Time: 30 minutes

Serving: 2

Size/ Portion: 1 piece

Ingredient:

- 1 tablespoon olive oil
- 1 cup cherry tomatoes
- 4 large fresh basil leaves, thinly sliced, divided
- 3 medium garlic cloves, minced
- 2 large portobello mushrooms, stems removed
- 4 pieces mini Mozzarella balls
- 1 tablespoon Parmesan cheese, grated

Direction:

1. Prep oven to 350°F (180°C). Grease a baking pan with olive oil.

2. Drizzle 1 tablespoon olive oil in a nonstick skillet, and heat over medium-high heat.

3. Add the tomatoes to the skillet, and sprinkle salt and black pepper to season. Prick some holes on the tomatoes for juice during the cooking. Put the lid on and cook the tomatoes for 10 minutes or until tender.

4. Reserve 2 teaspoons of basil and add the remaining basil and garlic to the skillet. Crush the tomatoes with a spatula, then cook for half a minute. Stir constantly during the cooking. Set aside.

5. Arrange the mushrooms in the baking pan, cap side down, and sprinkle with salt and black pepper to taste.

6. Spoon the tomato mixture and Mozzarella balls on the gill of the mushrooms, then scatter with Parmesan cheese to coat well.

7. Bake for 20 minutes

8. Remove the stuffed mushrooms from the oven and serve with basil on top.

Nutrition

285 calories

21.8g fat

14.3g protein

106.   Mushroom and Cheese Stuffed Tomatoes

Difficulty: Intermediate level

Preparation Time: 15 minutes

Cooking Time: 20 minutes

Serving: 4

Size/ Portion: 1 piece

Ingredients:

- 4 large ripe tomatoes
- 1 tablespoon olive oil
- ½ pound (454 g) white or cremini mushrooms
- 1 tablespoon fresh basil, chopped
- ½ cup yellow onion, diced
- 1 tablespoon fresh oregano, chopped
- 2 garlic cloves, minced
- ½ teaspoon salt
- ¼ teaspoon freshly ground black pepper
- 1 cup part-skim Mozzarella cheese, shredded
- 1 tablespoon Parmesan cheese, grated

Direction:

1. Set oven to 375°F (190°C).

2. Chop a ½-inch slice off the top of each tomato. Scoop the pulp into a bowl and leave ½-inch tomato shells. Arrange the tomatoes on a baking sheet lined with aluminum foil.

3. Heat the olive oil in a nonstick skillet over medium heat.

4. Add the mushrooms, basil, onion, oregano, garlic, salt, and black pepper to the skillet and sauté for 5 minutes

5. Pour the mixture to the bowl of tomato pulp, then add the Mozzarella cheese and stir to combine well.

6. Spoon the mixture into each tomato shell, then top with a layer of Parmesan.

7. Bake for 15 minutes

8. Remove the stuffed tomatoes from the oven and serve warm.

Nutrition:

254 calories

14.7g fat

17.5g protein

107. Tabbouleh

Difficulty: Intermediate level

Preparation Time: 15 minutes

Cooking Time: 5 minutes

Serving: 6

Size/ Portion: 2 cups

Ingredients:

- 4 tablespoons olive oil

- 4 cups riced cauliflower

- 3 garlic cloves

- ½ large cucumber

- ½ cup Italian parsley

- Juice of 1 lemon

- 2 tablespoons red onion

- ½ cup mint leaves, chopped

- ½ cup pitted Kalamata olives

- 1 cup cherry tomatoes

- 2 cups baby arugula

- 2 medium avocados

Direction:

1. Warm 2 tablespoons olive oil in a nonstick skillet over medium-high heat.

2. Add the rice cauliflower, garlic, salt, and black pepper to the skillet and sauté for 3 minutes or until fragrant. Transfer them to a large bowl.

3. Add the cucumber, parsley, lemon juice, red onion, mint, olives, and remaining olive oil to the bowl. Toss to combine well. Reserve the bowl in the refrigerator for at least 30 minutes.

4. Remove the bowl from the refrigerator. Add the cherry tomatoes, arugula, and avocado to the bowl. Sprinkle with salt and black pepper, and toss to combine well. Serve chilled.

Nutrition:

198 calories

17.5g fat

4.2g protein

108. Spicy Broccoli Rabe and Artichoke Hearts

Difficulty: Intermediate level

Preparation Time: 5 minutes

Cooking Time: 15 minutes

Serving: 4

Size/ Portion: ½ lb.

Ingredient:

- 3 tablespoons olive oil, divided
- 2 pounds fresh broccoli rabe
- 3 garlic cloves, finely minced
- 1 teaspoon red pepper flakes
- 1 teaspoon salt, plus more to taste
- 13.5 ounces artichoke hearts
- 1 tablespoon water
- 2 tablespoons red wine vinegar

Direction:

1. Warm 2 tablespoons olive oil in a nonstick skillet over medium-high skillet.

2. Add the broccoli, garlic, red pepper flakes, and salt to the skillet and sauté for 5 minutes or until the broccoli is soft.

3. Add the artichoke hearts to the skillet and sauté for 2 more minutes or until tender.

4. Add water to the skillet and turn down the heat to low. Put the lid on and simmer for 5 minutes.

5. Meanwhile, combine the vinegar and 1 tablespoon of olive oil in a bowl.

6. Drizzle the simmered broccoli and artichokes with oiled vinegar, and sprinkle with salt and black pepper. Toss to combine well before serving.

Nutrition:

272 calories

21.5g fat

11.2g protein

109. Shakshuka

Difficulty: Intermediate level

Preparation Time: 10 minutes

Cooking Time: 25 minutes

Serving: 4

Size/ portion: 1 cup

Ingredient:

- 5 tablespoons olive oil, divided
- 1 red bell pepper, finely diced
- ½ small yellow onion, finely diced
- 14 ounces crushed tomatoes, with juices
- 6 ounces frozen spinach
- 1 teaspoon smoked paprika
- 2 garlic cloves
- 2 teaspoons red pepper flakes
- 1 tablespoon capers
- 1 tablespoon water
- 6 large eggs
- ¼ teaspoon freshly ground black pepper
- ¾ cup feta or goat cheese
- ¼ cup fresh flat-leaf parsley

Direction:

1. Prep oven to 300°F (150°C).

2. Cook 2 tablespoons olive oil in an oven-safe skillet over medium-high heat.

3. Cook bell pepper and onion to the skillet for 6 minutes.

4. Add the tomatoes and juices, spinach, paprika, garlic, red pepper flakes, capers, water, and 2 tablespoons olive oil to the skillet. Stir and boil.

5. Turn down the heat to low, then put the lid on and simmer for 5 minutes.

6. Crack the eggs over the sauce, and keep a little space between each egg, leave the egg intact and sprinkle with freshly ground black pepper.

7. Cook for another 8 minutes

8. Scatter the cheese over the eggs and sauce, and bake in the preheated oven for 5 minutes

9. Drizzle 1 tablespoon olive oil and spread the parsley on top before serving warm.

Nutrition:

335 calories

26.5g fat

16.8g protein

110.   Spanakopita

Difficulty: Intermediate level

Preparation Time: 15 minutes

Cooking Time: 50 minutes

Serving: 6

Size/ Portion: 1 cup

Ingredients:

- 6 tablespoons olive oil
- 1 small yellow onion
- 4 cups frozen chopped spinach
- 4 garlic cloves, minced
- ½ teaspoon salt
- ½ teaspoon freshly ground black pepper
- 4 large eggs, beaten
- 1 cup ricotta cheese
- ¾ cup feta cheese, crumbled
- ¼ cup pine nuts

Direction

1. Set oven to 375°F (190°C). Coat a baking dish with 2 tablespoons olive oil.

2. Heat 2 tablespoons olive oil in a nonstick skillet over medium-high heat.

3. Add the onion to the skillet and sauté for 6 minutes or until translucent and tender.

4. Add the spinach, garlic, salt, and black pepper to the skillet and sauté for 5 minutes more. Keep aside

5. Combine the beaten eggs and ricotta cheese in a separate bowl, then pour them in to the bowl of spinach mixture. Stir to mix well.

6. Pour the mixture into the baking dish, and tilt the dish so the mixture coats the bottom evenly.

7. Bake for 20 minutes. Remove the baking dish from the oven, and spread the feta cheese and pine nuts on top, then drizzle with remaining 2 tablespoons olive oil.

8. Return the baking dish to the oven and bake for another 15 minutes

9. Remove the dish from the oven. Allow the spanakopita to cool for a few minutes and slice to serve.

Nutrition:

340 calories

27.3g fat

18.2g protein

111. Tagine

Difficulty: Intermediate level

Preparation Time: 20 minutes

Cooking Time: 1 hour

Serving: 6

Size/ Portion: 1 cup

Ingredients:

- ½ cup olive oil
- 6 celery stalks
- 2 medium yellow onions
- 1 teaspoon ground cumin

- ½ teaspoon ground cinnamon
- 1 teaspoon ginger powder
- 6 garlic cloves, minced
- ½ teaspoon paprika
- 1 teaspoon salt
- ¼ teaspoon freshly ground black pepper
- 2 cups low-sodium vegetable stock
- 2 medium zucchinis
- 2 cups cauliflower, cut into florets
- 1 medium eggplant
- 1 cup green olives
- 13.5 ounces artichoke hearts
- ½ cup chopped fresh cilantro leaves, for garnish
- ½ cup plain Greek yogurt, for garnish
- ½ cup chopped fresh flat-leaf parsley, for garnish

Direction:

1. Cook olive oil in a stockpot over medium-high heat.

2. Add the celery and onion to the pot and sauté for 6 minutes or until the celery is tender and the onion is translucent.

3. Add the cumin, cinnamon, ginger, garlic, paprika, salt, and black pepper to the pot and sauté for 2 minutes more until aromatic.

4. Pour the vegetable stock to the pot and bring to a boil.

5. Turn down the heat to low, and add the zucchini, cauliflower, and eggplant to the pot. Put the lid on and simmer for 30 minutes or until the vegetables are soft.

6. Then add the olives and artichoke hearts to the pot and simmer for 15 minutes more.

7. Pour them into a large serving bowl or a Tagine, then serve with cilantro, Greek yogurt, and parsley on top.

Nutrition

312 calories

21.2g fat

6.1g protein

112. Citrus Pistachios and Asparagus

Difficulty: Intermediate level

Preparation Time: 10 minutes

Cooking Time: 10 minutes

Serving: 4

Size/ Portion:

Ingredients:

- Zest and juice of 2 clementine
- Zest and juice of 1 lemon
- 1 tablespoon red wine vinegar
- 3 tablespoons extra-virgin olive oil
- 1 teaspoon salt
- ¼ teaspoon black pepper
- ½ cup pistachios, shelled
- 1-pound fresh asparagus
- 1 tablespoon water

Direction:

1. Combine the zest and juice of clementine and lemon, vinegar, 2 tablespoons of olive oil, ½ teaspoon of salt, and black pepper in a bowl. Stir to mix well. Set aside.

2. Toast the pistachios in a nonstick skillet over medium-high heat for 2 minutes or until golden brown. Transfer the roasted pistachios to a clean work surface, then chop roughly. Mix the pistachios with the citrus mixture. Set aside.

3. Heat the remaining olive oil in the nonstick skillet over medium-high heat.

4. Add the asparagus to the skillet and sauté for 2 minutes, then season with remaining salt.

5. Add the water to the skillet. Turn down the heat to low, and put the lid on. Simmer for 4 minutes until the asparagus is tender.

6. Remove the asparagus from the skillet to a large dish. Pour the citrus and pistachios mixture over the asparagus. Toss to coat well before serving.

Nutrition:

211 calories

17.5g fat

5.9g protein

113. Tomato and Parsley Stuffed Eggplant

Difficulty: Intermediate level

Preparation Time: 25 minutes

Cooking Time: 2 hours

Serving: 6

Size/ portion: ½ cup

Ingredients:

- ¼ cup extra-virgin olive oil
- 3 small eggplants, cut in half lengthwise
- 1 teaspoon sea salt
- ½ teaspoon freshly ground black pepper
- 1 large yellow onion, finely chopped
- 4 garlic cloves, minced
- 15 ounces diced tomatoes
- ¼ cup fresh flat-leaf parsley

Direction:

1. Brush inserts of the slow cooker with 2 tablespoons of olive oil.

2. Cut some slits on the cut side of each eggplant half, keep a ¼-inch space between each slit.

3. Place the eggplant halves in the slow cooker, skin side down. Sprinkle with salt and black pepper.

4. Cook remaining olive oil in a nonstick skillet over medium-high heat.

5. Add the onion and garlic to the skillet and sauté for 3 minutes or until the onion is translucent.

6. Add the parsley and tomatoes with the juice to the skillet, and sprinkle with salt and black pepper. Sauté for 5 more minutes or until they are tender.

7. Divide and spoon the mixture in the skillet on the eggplant halves.

8. Close and cook on HIGH for 2 hours.

9. Transfer the eggplant to a plate, and allow to cool for a few minutes before serving.

Nutrition:

455 calories

13g fat

14g protein

114. Ratatouille

Difficulty: Professional level

Preparation Time: 15 minutes

Cooking Time: 7 hours

Serving: 6

Size/ Portion: 2 ounces

Ingredient:

- 3 tablespoons extra-virgin olive oil
- 1 large eggplant

- 2 large onions
- 4 small zucchinis
- 2 green bell peppers
- 6 large tomatoes
- 2 tablespoons fresh flat-leaf parsley
- 1 teaspoon dried basil
- 2 garlic cloves, minced
- 2 teaspoons sea salt
- ¼ teaspoon black pepper

Direction

1. Grease inserts of the slow cooker with 2 tablespoons olive oil.

2. Arrange the vegetables slices, strips, and wedges alternately in the insert of the slow cooker.

3. Spread the parsley on top of the vegetables, and season with basil, garlic, salt, and black pepper. Drizzle with the remaining olive oil.

4. Cover on and cook on LOW for 7 hours until the vegetables are tender.

5. Transfer the vegetables on a plate and serve warm.

Nutrition:

265 calories

1.7g fat

8.3g protein

115.   Gemista

Difficulty: Professional level

Preparation Time: 15 minutes

Cooking Time: 4 hours

Serving: 4

Size/ portion: 2 ounces

Ingredients:

- 2 tablespoons extra-virgin olive oil
- 4 large bell peppers, any color
- ½ cup uncooked couscous
- 1 teaspoon oregano
- 1 garlic clove, minced
- 1 cup crumbled feta cheese
- 1 (15-ounce) can cannellini beans
- 4 green onions

Direction:

1. Brush inserts of the slow cooker with 2 tablespoons olive oil.

2. Cut a ½-inch slice below the stem from the top of the bell pepper. Discard the stem only and chop the sliced top portion under the stem, and reserve in a bowl. Hollow the bell pepper with a spoon.

3. Mix remaining ingredients, except for the green parts of the green onion and lemon wedges, to the bowl of chopped bell pepper top. Stir to mix well.

4. Spoon the mixture in the hollowed bell pepper, and arrange the stuffed bell peppers in the slow cooker, then drizzle with more olive oil.

5. Close and cook at HIGH for 4 hours or until the bell peppers are soft.

6. Remove the bell peppers from the slow cooker and serve on a plate. Sprinkle with green parts of the green onions, and squeeze the lemon wedges on top before serving.

Nutrition:

246 calories

9g fat

11.1g protein

116.   Stuffed Cabbage Rolls

Difficulty: Professional level

Preparation Time: 15 minutes

Cooking Time: 2 hours

Serving: 4

Size/ Portion: 1 roll

Ingredients:

- 4 tablespoons olive oil
- 1 large head green cabbage
- 1 large yellow onion
- 3 ounces (85 g) feta cheese
- ½ cup dried currants
- 3 cups cooked pearl barley
- 2 tablespoons fresh flat-leaf parsley
- 2 tablespoons pine nuts, toasted
- ½ teaspoon sea salt
- ½ teaspoon black pepper
- 15 ounces (425 g) crushed tomatoes, with the juice
- ½ cup apple juice
- 1 tablespoon apple cider vinegar

Direction:

1. Rub insert of the slow cooker with 2 tablespoons olive oil.

2. Blanch the cabbage in a pot of water for 8 minutes. Remove it from the water, and allow to cool, then separate 16 leaves from the cabbage. Set aside.

3. Drizzle the remaining olive oil in a nonstick skillet, and heat over medium heat.

4. Sauté onion for 6 minutes. Transfer the onion to a bowl.

5. Add the feta cheese, currants, barley, parsley, and pine nuts to the bowl of cooked onion, then sprinkle with ¼ teaspoon of salt and ¼ teaspoon of black pepper.

6. Arrange the cabbage leaves on a clean work surface. Spoon 1/3 cup of the mixture on the center of each leaf, then fold the edge of the leaf over the mixture and roll it up. Place the cabbage rolls in the slow cooker, seam side down.

7. Combine the remaining ingredients in a separate bowl, then pour the mixture over the cabbage rolls.

8. Close and cook in HIGH for 2 hours.

9. Remove the cabbage rolls from the slow cooker and serve warm.

Nutrition:

383 calories

17g fat

11g protein

117.   Brussels Sprouts with Balsamic Glaze

Difficulty: Professional level

Preparation Time: 15 minutes

Cooking Time: 2 hours

Serving: 6

Size/ Portion: 1 lb.

Balsamic glaze:

- 1 cup balsamic vinegar
- ¼ cup honey

Other:

- 2 tablespoons extra-virgin olive oil
- 2 pounds (907 g) Brussels sprouts
- 2 cups low-sodium vegetable soup
- 1 teaspoon sea salt

- Freshly ground black pepper, to taste
- ¼ cup Parmesan cheese, grated
- ¼ cup pine nuts, toasted

Direction:

1. Brush inserts of the slow cooker with olive oil.

2. Make the balsamic glaze: Combine the balsamic vinegar and honey in a saucepan. Stir to mix well. Over medium-high heat, bring to a boil. Turn down the heat to low, then simmer for 20 minutes or until the glaze reduces in half and has a thick consistency.

3. Put the Brussels sprouts, vegetable soup, and ½ teaspoon of salt in the slow cooker, stir to combine.

4. Cover and cook at HIGH for 2 hours.

5. Transfer the Brussels sprouts to a plate, and sprinkle the remaining salt and black pepper to season. Drizzle the balsamic glaze over the Brussels sprouts, then serve with Parmesan and pine nuts.

Nutrition:

270 calories

11g fat

8.7g protein

118. Spinach Salad with Citrus Vinaigrette

Difficulty: Professional level

Preparation Time: 10 minutes

Cooking Time: 0 minutes

Servings: 4

Size/ portion: 2 cups

Ingredients:

Citrus Vinaigrette:

- ¼ cup extra-virgin olive oil

- 3 tablespoons balsamic vinegar
- ½ teaspoon fresh lemon zest
- ½ teaspoon salt

SALAD:

- 1-pound (454 g) baby spinach
- 1 large ripe tomato
- 1 medium red onion

Direction:

1. Make the citrus vinaigrette: Stir together the olive oil, balsamic vinegar, lemon zest, and salt in a bowl until mixed well.

2. Make the salad: Place the baby spinach, tomato and onions in a separate salad bowl. Drizzle the citrus vinaigrette over the salad and gently toss until the vegetables are coated thoroughly.

Nutrition:

173 Calories

14g fat

4.1g protein

119. Kale Salad with Pistachio and Parmesan

Difficulty: Professional level

Preparation Time: 20 minutes

Cooking Time: 0 minutes

Serving: 6

Size/ Portion: 2 cups

Ingredients:

- 6 cups raw kale
- ¼ cup extra-virgin olive oil
- 2 tablespoons lemon juice
- ½ teaspoon smoked paprika
- 2 cups chopped arugula

- 1/3 cup unsalted pistachios

- 6 tablespoons Parmesan cheese

Direction:

1. Put the kale, olive oil, lemon juice, and paprika in a large bowl. Using your hands to massage the sauce into the kale until coated completely. Allow the kale to marinate for about 10 minutes.

2. When ready to serve, add the arugula and pistachios into the bowl of kale. Toss well and divide the salad into six salad bowls. Serve sprinkled with 1 tablespoon shredded Parmesan cheese.

Nutrition:

106 Calories

9.2g fat

4.2g protein

120. Israeli Eggplant, Chickpea, and Mint Sauté

Difficulty: Intermediate level

Preparation Time: 5 minutes

Cooking Time: 20 minutes

Serving: 6

Size/ Portion: 2 cups

Ingredients:

- 1 medium globe eggplant

- 1 tablespoon extra-virgin olive oil

- 2 tablespoons lemon juice

- 2 tablespoons balsamic vinegar

- 1 teaspoon ground cumin

- ¼ teaspoon salt

- 1 (15-ounce) can chickpeas

- 1 cup sliced sweet onion

- ¼ cup mint leaves

- 1 tablespoon sesame seeds

- 1 garlic clove

Direction:

1. Place one oven rack about 4 inches below the broiler element. Turn the broiler to the highest setting to preheat. Grease rimmed baking sheet using nonstick cooking spray.

2. Slice eggplant lengthwise into four slabs (½- to 5/8-inch thick). Place the eggplant slabs on the prepared baking sheet. Put aside.

3. Scourge oil, lemon juice, vinegar, cumin, and salt. Brush 2 tablespoons of the lemon dressing over both sides of the eggplant slabs.

4. Broil the eggplant under the heating element for 4 minutes, flip them, and then broil for 4 minutes.

5. While the eggplant is broiling, combine the chickpeas, onion, mint, sesame seeds, and garlic. Add the reserved dressing, and gently mix.

6. When done, situate slabs from the baking sheet to a cooling rack and cool for 3 minutes. When slightly cooled, cut each slab crosswise into ½-inch strips.

7. Toss eggplant to the mixture and serve warm.

Nutrition:

159 Calories

4g Fat

6g Protein

121. Mediterranean Lentils and Rice

Difficulty: Professional level

Preparation Time: 5 minutes

Cooking Time: 25 minutes

Serving: 4

Size/ Portion: 2 cups

Ingredients:

- 2¼ cups low-sodium vegetable broth
- ½ cup lentils
- ½ cup uncooked instant brown rice
- ½ cup diced carrots
- ½ cup diced celery
- 1 (2.25-ounce) can sliced olives
- ¼ cup diced red onion
- ¼ cup chopped fresh curly-leaf parsley
- 1½ tablespoons extra-virgin olive oil
- 1 tablespoon freshly squeezed lemon juice
- 1 garlic clove
- ¼ teaspoon kosher or sea salt
- ¼ teaspoon black pepper

Direction:

1. Position saucepan over high heat, bring the broth and lentils to a boil, cover, and lower the heat to medium-low. Cook for 8 minutes.

2. Raise the heat to medium, and stir in the rice. Cover the pot and cook the mixture for 15 minutes. Take away pot from the heat and let it sit, covered, for 1 minute, then stir.

3. While the lentils and rice are cooking, mix together the carrots, celery, olives, onion, and parsley in a large serving bowl.

4. In a small bowl, whisk together the oil, lemon juice, garlic, salt, and pepper. Set aside.

5. When cooked, put them to the serving bowl. Pour the dressing on top, and mix everything together. Serve.

Nutrition:

230 Calories

8g Fat

8g Protein

122. Brown Rice Pilaf with Golden Raisins

Difficulty: Professional level

Preparation Time: 5 minutes

Cooking Time: 15 minutes

Serving: 6

Size/ Portion: 2 cups

Ingredients:

- 1 tablespoon extra-virgin olive oil
- 1 cup chopped onion
- ½ cup shredded carrot
- 1 teaspoon ground cumin
- ½ teaspoon ground cinnamon
- 2 cups instant brown rice
- 1¾ cups 100% orange juice
- ¼ cup water
- 1 cup golden raisins
- ½ cup shelled pistachios

Direction:

1. Put saucepan on medium-high heat, cook onion for 5 minutes. Sauté carrot, cumin, and cinnamon.

2. Stir in the rice, orange juice, and water. Bring to a boil, cover, then lower the heat to medium-low. Simmer for 7 minutes.

3. Stir in the raisins, pistachios, and chives (if using) and serve.

Nutrition:

320 Calories

7g Fat

6g Protein

123. Chinese Soy Eggplant

Difficulty: Intermediate level

Preparation Time: 5 Minutes

Cooking Time: 10 Minutes

Servings: 2

Ingredients:

- Four tablespoons coconut oil
- Two eggplants, sliced into 3-inch in length
- Four cloves of garlic, minced
- One onion, chopped
- One teaspoon ginger, grated
- ¼ cup coconut aminos
- One teaspoon lemon juice, freshly squeezed

Directions:

1. Heat oil in a pot.
2. Pan-fry the eggplants for minutes on all sides.
3. Add the garlic and onions until fragrant, around minutes.
4. Stir in the ginger, coconut aminos, and lemon juice.
5. Add a ½ cup of water and let it simmer. Cook until eggplant is tender.

Nutrition:

Calories per **Serving:** 409

Carbs: 40.8g

Protein: 6.6g

Fat: 28.3g

124. Cauliflower Mash

Difficulty: Intermediate level

Preparation Time: 5 Minutes

Cooking Time: 0 Minutes

Servings: 2

Ingredients:

- Crushed red pepper to taste
- 1 tsp fresh thyme
- 2 tsp chopped chives
- 2 tbsp. **Nutritional** yeast
- 2 tbsp. filtered water
- One garlic clove, peeled
- One lemon, juice extracted
- ¼ cup pine nuts
- 3 cups cauliflower, chopped

Directions:

1. Mix all fixings in a blender or food processor. Pulse until smooth.
2. Scoop into a bowl and add crushed red peppers.

Nutrition:

Calories per **Serving:** 224

Carbs: 19.8g

Protein: 10.5g

Fat: 13.6g

125. Vegetarian Cabbage Rolls

Difficulty: Intermediate level

Preparation Time: 5 Minutes

Cooking Time: 1 Hour and 30 Minutes

Servings: 2

Ingredients:

- One large head green cabbage
- 1 cup long-grain rice, rinsed
- Two medium zucchinis, finely diced
- 4 TB. minced garlic
- 2 tsp. salt
- 1 tsp. ground black pepper
- 4 cups plain tomato sauce
- 2 cups of water
- 1 tsp. dried mint

Directions:

1. Cut around a core of cabbage with a knife, and remove the core. Put cabbage, with core side down, in a large, 3-quart pot. Cover cabbage with water, set over high heat, and cook for 30 minutes. Drain cabbage, set aside to cool, and separate leaves. (You need 24 leaves.)

2. In a large bowl, combine long-grain rice, zucchini, one tablespoon garlic, one teaspoon salt, and 1/teaspoon black pepper.
3. In a 2-quart pot, combine tomato sauce, water, remaining tablespoons garlic, mint, remaining one teaspoon salt, and 1/2 teaspoon black pepper.
4. Lay each cabbage leaf flat on your work surface, spoon two tablespoons filling each leaf, and roll leaf. Layer rolls in a large pot, pour the sauce into the pot, cover, and cook over medium-low heat for 1 hour.
5. Let rolls sit for 20 minutes before serving warm with Greek yogurt.

Nutrition:

Calories per **Serving:** 120

Carbs: 8.0g

Protein: 2.3g

Fat: 9.5g

126. Vegan Sesame Tofu and Eggplants

Difficulty: Intermediate level

Preparation Time: 5 Minutes

Cooking Time: 15 Minutes

Servings: 4

Ingredients:

- Five tablespoons olive oil
- 1-pound firm tofu, sliced
- Three tablespoons rice vinegar
- Two teaspoons Swerve sweetener
- Two whole eggplants, sliced
- ¼ cup of soy sauce
- Salt and pepper to taste
- Four tablespoons toasted sesame oil
- ¼ cup sesame seeds
- 1 cup fresh cilantro, chopped

Directions:

1. Heat the oil in a pan for 2 minutes.
2. Pan-fry the tofu for 3 minutes on each side.

3. Stir in the rice vinegar, sweetener, eggplants, and soy sauce—season with salt and pepper to taste.
4. Close the lid, then cook for around 5 minutes on medium fire. Stir and continue cooking for another 5 minutes.
5. Toss in the sesame oil, sesame seeds, and cilantro.
6. Serve and enjoy.

Nutrition:

Calories per **Serving:** 616

Carbs: 27.4g

Protein: 23.9g

Fat: 49.2g

127. Steamed Squash Chowder

Difficulty: Intermediate level

Preparation Time: 5 Minutes

Cooking Time: 40 Minutes

Servings: 4

Ingredients:

- 3 cups chicken broth
- 2 tbsp. ghee
- 1 tsp chili powder
- ½ tsp cumin
- 1 ½ tsp salt
- 2 tsp cinnamon
- 3 tbsp. olive oil
- Two carrots, chopped
- One small yellow onion, chopped
- One green apple, sliced and cored
- One large butternut squash

Directions:

1. In a large pot on medium-high fire, melt ghee.
2. Once the ghee is hot, sauté onions for 5 minutes or until soft and translucent.
3. Add olive oil, chili powder, cumin, salt, and cinnamon. Sauté for half a minute.
4. Add chopped squash and apples.
5. Sauté for 10 minutes while stirring once in a while.

6. Add broth, cover, and cook on medium fire for twenty minutes or until apples and squash are tender.
7. With an immersion blender, puree the chowder. Adjust consistency by adding more water.
8. Add more salt or pepper depending on desire.
9. Serve and enjoy.

Nutrition:

Calories per **Serving:** 228

Carbs: 17.9g

Protein: 2.2g

Fat: 18.0g

128.   Collard Green Wrap Greek Style

Difficulty: Professional level

Preparation Time: 5 Minutes

Cooking Time: 0 Minutes

Servings: 4

Ingredients:

- ½ block feta, cut into 4 (1-inch thick) strips (4-oz)
- ½ cup purple onion, diced
- ½ medium red bell pepper, julienned
- One medium cucumber, julienned
- Four large cherry tomatoes halved
- Four large collard green leaves washed
- Eight whole kalamata olives halved
- 1 cup full-fat plain Greek yogurt
- One tablespoon white vinegar
- One teaspoon garlic powder
- Two tablespoons minced fresh dill
- Two tablespoons olive oil
- 2.5-ounces cucumber, seeded and grated (¼-whole)
- Salt and pepper to taste

Directions:

1. Make the Tzatziki sauce first: make sure to squeeze out all the excess liquid from the cucumber after grating. In a small bowl, mix all sauce fixings thoroughly and refrigerate.
2. Prepare and slice all wrap ingredients.
3. On a flat surface, spread one collard green leaf. Spread two tablespoons of Tzatziki sauce in the middle of the leaf.
4. Layer ¼ of each of the tomatoes, feta, olives, onion, pepper, and cucumber. Place them on the center of the leaf, like piling them high instead of spreading them.
5. Fold the leaf like you would a burrito. Repeat process for remaining ingredients.
6. Serve and enjoy.

Nutrition:

Calories per **Serving:** 165.3

Protein: 7.0g

Carbs: 9.9g

Fat: 11.2g

129.   Cayenne Eggplant Spread

Difficulty: Professional level

Preparation Time: 5 Minutes

Cooking Time: 50 Minutes

Servings: 4

Ingredients:

- Two eggplants, trimmed
- One teaspoon cayenne pepper
- One teaspoon salt
- ½ teaspoon harissa
- One tablespoon sesame oil
- Three tablespoons Plain yogurt
- One garlic clove, peeled
- 1/3 teaspoon sumac
- One teaspoon ground paprika
- One teaspoon lemon juice

Directions:

1. Cut the eggplants on the halves and rub them with salt.
2. Preheat the oven to 375F.
3. Arrange the eggplant halves in the tray and bake them for 50 minutes.

4. When the eggplants are soft, they are ready to be used.
5. Peel the eggplants and put the peeled eggplant pulp in the blender.
6. Add cayenne pepper, harissa, sesame oil, Plain yogurt, garlic clove, sumac, and lemon juice.
7. Blend the mixture until smooth and soft.
8. Transfer the cooked meal to the serving bowls and sprinkle with ground paprika.

Nutrition:

Calories 113

Fat 4.3

Fiber 10

Carbs 18

Protein 3.6

130.   Cilantro Potato Mash

Difficulty: Professional level

Preparation Time: 5 Minutes

Cooking Time: 20 Minutes

Servings: 2

Ingredients:

- 1 cup yam, chopped
- One tablespoon cream
- ½ teaspoon dried cilantro
- 1 cup of water
- ½ teaspoon salt

Directions:

1. Boil yum in water for 20 minutes or until it is soft.
2. Then drain the water and mash the yam with the help of the potato masher.
3. Add cream dried cilantro, and salt.
4. Mix up well.

Nutrition:

Calories 92

Fat 0.5

Fiber 3.1

Carbs 21.1

Protein 1.2

131.   Cheese and Broccoli Balls

Difficulty: Professional level

Preparation Time: 5 Minutes

Cooking Time: 5 Minutes

Servings: 4

Ingredients:

- ¾ cup almond flour
- Two large eggs
- Two teaspoons baking powder
- 4 ounces fresh broccoli
- 4 ounces mozzarella cheese
- Seven tablespoons flaxseed meal
- Salt and Pepper to taste
- ¼ cup fresh chopped dill
- ¼ cup mayonnaise
- ½ tablespoon lemon juice
- Salt and pepper to taste

Directions:

1. Place broccoli in the food processor and pulse into small pieces. Transfer to a bowl.
2. Add ¼ cup flaxseed meal, baking powder, almond flour, and cheese. Season with pepper and salt if desired. Mix well— place remaining flaxseed meal in a small bowl.
3. Add eggs and combine thoroughly. Roll the batter into 1-inch balls. Then roll in flaxseed meal to hide the balls.
4. Cook balls in a 375oF deep-fryer until golden brown, about 5 minutes. Transfer cooked balls on to a paper towel-lined plate.
5. In the meantime, make the sauce by combining all fixings in a medium bowl.
6. Serve cheese and broccoli balls with the plunging sauce on the side.

Nutrition:

Calories per **Serving:** 312

Protein: 18.4g

Carbs: 9.6g

Fat: 23.2g

132.   Hot Pepper Sauce

Difficulty: Professional level

Preparation Time: 10 Minutes

Cooking Time: 20 Minutes

Servings: 4 Cups

Ingredients:

- Two red hot fresh chiles, deseeded
- Two dried chiles
- Two garlic cloves, peeled
- ½ small yellow onion, roughly chopped
- 2 cups of water
- 2 cups white vinegar

Directions:

1. Place all the fixings except the vinegar in a medium saucepan over medium heat. Allow simmering for 20 minutes until softened.
2. Transfer the combination to a food processor or blender. Stir in the vinegar and pulse until very smooth.
3. Serve instantly or transfer to a sealed container and refrigerate for up to 3 months.

Nutrition:

Calories: 20

Fat: 1.2g

Protein: 0.6g

Carbs: 4.4g

Fiber: 0.6g

Sodium: 12mg

133.   Avocado Gazpacho

Difficulty: Professional level

Preparation Time: 15 minutes

Cooking Time: 0 minute

Serving: 4

Size/ portion: 2 cups

Ingredients:

- 2 cups chopped tomatoes
- 2 large ripe avocados
- 1 large cucumber
- 1 medium bell pepper
- 1 cup plain whole-milk Greek yogurt
- ¼ cup extra-virgin olive oil
- ¼ cup chopped fresh cilantro
- ¼ cup chopped scallions
- 2 tablespoons red wine vinegar
- Juice of 2 limes or 1 lemon
- ½ to 1 teaspoon salt
- ¼ teaspoon black pepper

Direction:

1. In a blender or in a large bowl, if using an immersion blender, combine the tomatoes, avocados, cucumber, bell pepper, yogurt, olive oil, and cilantro, scallions, vinegar, and lime juice. Blend until smooth. If using a stand blender, you may need to blend in two or three batches.
2. Season with salt and pepper and blend to combine the flavors.
3. Chill for 2 hours before serving. Serve cold.

Nutrition:

392 Calories

32g Fat

6g Protein

134.   Roasted Garlic Hummus

Difficulty: Professional level

Preparation Time: 9 minutes

Cooking Time: 33 minutes

Serving: 4

Size/ Portion: 2 tablespoons

Ingredients:

- 1 cup dried chickpeas
- 4 cups water
- 1 tablespoon plus ¼ cup extra-virgin olive oil, divided
- 1/3 cup tahini
- 1 teaspoon ground cumin
- ½ teaspoon onion powder
- ¾ teaspoon salt
- ½ teaspoon ground black pepper
- 1/3 cup lemon juice
- 3 tablespoons mashed roasted garlic
- 2 tablespoons chopped fresh parsley

Direction:

1. Situate chickpeas, water, and 1 tablespoon oil in the Instant Pot®. Cover, press steam release to Sealing, set Manual button, and time to 30 minutes.

2. When the timer beeps, quick-release the pressure. Select Cancel button and open. Strain, reserving the cooking liquid.

3. Place chickpeas, remaining ¼ cup oil, tahini, cumin, onion powder, salt, pepper, lemon juice, and roasted garlic in a food processor and process until creamy. Top with parsley. Serve at room temperature.

Nutrition

104 Calories

6g Fat

4g Protein

Seafood

135. Pistachio-Crusted Whitefish

Preparation Time: 10 minutes

Cooking Time: 20 minutes

Servings: 2

Ingredients:

- ¼ cup shelled pistachios
- 1 tbsp. fresh parsley
- 1 tbsp. grated Parmesan cheese
- 1 tbsp. panko bread crumbs
- 2 tbsps. olive oil
- ¼ tsp. salt
- 10 oz. skinless whitefish (1 large piece or 2 smaller ones)

Directions:

1. Preheat the oven to 350°F and set the rack to the middle position. Line a sheet pans with foil or parchment paper.
2. Combine all of the ingredients except the fish in a mini food processor and pulse until the nuts are finely ground.
3. Alternatively, you can mince the nuts with a chef's knife and combine the ingredients by hand in a small bowl.
4. Place the fish on the sheet pan. Spread the nut mixture evenly over the fish and pat it down lightly.
5. Bake the fish for 20 to 30 minutes, depending on the thickness, until it flakes easily with a fork.
6. Keep in mind that a thicker cut of fish takes a bit longer to bake. You'll know it's done when it's opaque, flakes apart easily with a fork, or reaches an internal temperature of 145°F.

Nutrition:

Calories: 185

Protein: 10.1g

Fats: 5.2g

Carbohydrates: 23.8g

136. Grilled Fish on Lemons

Preparation Time: 10 minutes

Cooking Time: 10 minutes

Servings: 2

Ingredients:

- 4 (4-oz.) fish fillets, such as tilapia, salmon, catfish, cod, or your favorite fish
- Nonstick cooking spray
- 3 to 4 medium lemons
- 1 tbsp. extra-virgin olive oil
- ¼ tsp. freshly ground black pepper
- ¼ tsp. kosher or sea salt

Directions:

1. Using paper towels pat the fillets dry and let stand at room temperature for 10 minutes.
2. Meanwhile, coat the cold cooking grate of the grill with nonstick cooking spray and preheat the grill to 400°F, or medium-high heat. Or preheat a grill pan over medium-high heat on the stovetop.
3. Cut 1 lemon in half and set half aside. Slice the remaining half of that lemon and the remaining lemons into ¼-inch-thick slices (You should have about 12 to 16 lemon slices).
4. Into a small bowl, squeeze 1 tablespoon of juice out of the reserved lemon half.
5. Add the oil to the bowl with the lemon juice and mix well.
6. Brush both sides of the fish with the oil mixture and sprinkle evenly with pepper and salt.
7. Carefully place the lemon slices on the grill (or the grill pan), arranging 3 to 4 slices together in the shape of a fish fillet and repeat with the remaining slices.
8. Place the fish fillets directly on top of the lemon slices and grill with the lid closed (If you're grilling on the stovetop, cover with a large pot lid or aluminum foil).
9. Turn the fish halfway through the cooking time only if the fillets are more than half an inch thick.

10. The fish is done and ready to serve when it just begins to separate into flakes (chunks) when pressed gently with a fork.

Nutrition:

Calories: 185

Protein: 10.1g

Fats: 5.2g

Carbohydrates: 23.8g

137. Weeknight Sheet Pan Fish Dinner

Preparation Time: 10 minutes

Cooking Time: 10 minutes

Servings: 2

Ingredients:

- Nonstick cooking spray
- 2 tbsps. extra-virgin olive oil
- 1 tbsp. balsamic vinegar
- 4 (4-oz.) fish fillets, such as cod or tilapia (½ inch thick)
- 2½ cup green beans (about 12 oz.)
- 1-pint cherry or grape tomatoes (about 2 cups)

Directions:

1. Preheat the oven to 400°F. Coat 2 large, rimmed baking sheets with nonstick cooking spray.
2. In a small bowl, whisk together the oil and vinegar. Set aside. Place 2 pieces of fish on each baking sheet.
3. In a large bowl, combine the beans and tomatoes. Pour in the oil and vinegar and toss gently to coat.
4. Pour half of the green bean mixture over the fish on 1 baking sheet and the remaining half over the fish on the other.
5. Turn the fish over and rub it in the oil mixture to coat. Spread the vegetables evenly on the baking sheets so hot air can circulate around them.
6. Bake for 5 to 8 minutes, until the fish is just opaque and not translucent. The fish is done and ready to serve when it just

begins to separate into flakes (chunks) when pressed gently with a fork.

Nutrition:

Calories: 185

Protein: 10.1g

Fats: 5.2g

Carbohydrates: 23.8g

138. Crispy Polenta Fish Sticks

Preparation Time: 15 minutes

Cooking Time: 10 minutes

Servings: 2

Ingredients:

- 2 large eggs, lightly beaten
- 1 tbsp. 2% milk
- 1 lb. skinned fish fillets (cod, tilapia, or other white fish) about ½ inch thick, sliced into 20 (1-inch-wide) strips
- ½ cup yellow cornmeal
- ½ cup whole-wheat panko bread crumbs or whole-wheat bread crumbs
- ¼ tsp. smoked paprika
- ¼ tsp. kosher or sea salt
- ¼ tsp. freshly ground black pepper
- Nonstick cooking spray

Directions:

1. Place a large, rimmed baking sheet in the oven. Preheat the oven to 400°F with the pan inside. In a large bowl, mix the eggs and milk.
2. Using a fork, add the fish strips to the egg mixture and stir gently to coat.
3. Put the cornmeal, bread crumbs, smoked paprika, salt and pepper in a quart-size zip-top plastic bag.
4. Using a fork or tongs, transfer the fish to the bag letting the excess egg wash drip off into the bowl before transferring. Seal the bag and shake gently to completely coat each fish stick.
5. With oven mitts, carefully remove the hot baking sheet from the oven and spray it with nonstick cooking spray.

6. Using a fork or tongs, remove the fish sticks from the bag and arrange them on the hot baking sheet, with space between them so the hot air can circulate and crisp them up.
7. Bake for 5 to 8 minutes, until gentle pressure with a fork causes the fish to flake and serve.

Nutrition:

Calories: 185

Protein: 10.1g

Fats: 5.2g

Carbohydrates: 23.8g

139. Crispy Homemade Fish Sticks Recipe

Preparation Time: 10 minutes

Cooking Time: 15 minutes

Servings: 2

Ingredients:

- ½ cup flour
- 1 beaten egg
- 1 cup flour
- ½ cup parmesan cheese
- ½ cup bread crumbs.
- 1 lemon juice zest
- Parsley
- Salt
- 1 tsp. black pepper
- 1 tbsp. sweet paprika
- 1 tsp. oregano
- 1½ lb. salmon
- Extra virgin olive oil

Directions:

1. Preheat your oven to about 450°F. Get a bowl, dry your salmon and season its 2 sides with the salt.
2. Then chop into small sizes of 1½-inch length each. Get a bowl and mix black pepper with oregano.
3. Add paprika to the mixture and blend it. Then spice the fish stick with the mixture

you have just made. Get another dish and pour your flour.
4. You will need a different bowl again to pour your egg wash into. Pick yet the fourth dish, mix your breadcrumb with your parmesan and add lemon zest to the mixture.
5. Return to the fish sticks and dip each fish into flour such that both sides are coated with flour. As you dip each fish into flour, take it out and dip it into the egg wash and lastly. Dip it in the breadcrumb mixture.
6. Do this for all fish sticks and arrange them on a baking sheet. Ensure you oil the baking sheet before arranging the stick thereon and drizzle the top of the fish sticks with extra virgin olive oil.

Caution: allow excess flours to fall off a fish before dipping it into other ingredients.

Also, ensure that you do not let the coating peel while you add extra virgin olive oil on top of the fishes.

Fix the baking sheet in the middle of the oven and allow it to cook for 13 minutes. By then, the fishes should be golden brown and you can retire them from the oven and you can serve them immediately.

Top it with your lemon zest, parsley and fresh lemon juice.

Nutrition:

Calories: 119

Protein: 13.5g

Fats: 3.4g

Carbohydrates: 9.3g

140. Sauced Shellfish in White Wine

Preparation Time: 10 minutes

Cooking Time: 10 minutes

Servings: 2

Ingredients:

- 2 lbs. fresh cuttlefish

- ½ cup olive oil
- 1 large onion, finely chopped
- 1 cup Robola white wine
- ¼ cup lukewarm water
- 1 bay leaf
- ½ bunch parsley, chopped
- 4 tomatoes, grated
- Salt and pepper

Directions:

1. Take out the hard centerpiece of cartilage (cuttlebone), the bag of ink and the intestines from the cuttlefish.
2. Wash the cleaned cuttlefish with running water. Slice it into small pieces and drain the excess water.
3. Heat the oil in a saucepan placed over medium-high heat and sauté the onion for 3 minutes until tender.
4. Add the sliced cuttlefish and pour in the white wine. Cook for 5 minutes until it simmers.
5. Pour in the water and add the tomatoes, bay leaf, parsley, tomatoes, salt and pepper. Simmer the mixture over low heat until the cuttlefish slices are tender and left with their thick sauce. Serve them warm with rice.
6. Be careful not to overcook the cuttlefish as its texture becomes very hard. A safe rule of thumb is grilling the cuttlefish over a ragingly hot fire for 3 minutes before using it in any recipe.

Nutrition:

Calories:3 08

Protein: 25.6g

Fats: 18.1g

Carbohydrates: 8g

141. Pistachio Sole Fish

Preparation Time: 5 minutes

Cooking Time: 10 minutes

Servings: 2

Ingredients:

- 4 (5 oz.) boneless sole fillets
- ½ cup pistachios, finely chopped
- 1 lemon juice
- 1 tsp. extra virgin olive oil

Directions:

1. Preheat your oven to 350°F.
2. Wrap a baking sheet using parchment paper and keep it on the side.
3. Pat fish dry with kitchen towels and lightly season with salt and pepper.
4. Take a small bowl and stir in the pistachios.
5. Place sole fillets on the prepped sheet and press 2 tablespoons of pistachio mixture on top of each fillet.
6. Rub the fish with lemon juice and olive oil.
7. Bake for 10 minutes until the top is golden and fish flakes with a fork.

Nutrition:

Calories:1 66

Protein 6g

Fats: 6g

Carbohydrates: 2g

142. Speedy Tilapia with Red Onion and Avocado

Preparation Time: 10 minutes

Cooking Time: 5 minutes

Servings: 2

Ingredients:

- 1 tbsp. extra-virgin olive oil
- 1 tbsp. freshly squeezed orange juice
- ¼ tsp. kosher or sea salt
- 4 (4-oz.) tilapia fillets, more oblong than square, skin-on or skinned
- ¼ cup chopped red onion (about 1/8 onion)
- 1 avocado, pitted, skinned, and sliced

Directions:

1. In a 9-inch glass pie dish, use a fork to mix together the oil, orange juice and salt. Working with 1 fillet at a time, place each in the pie dish and turn to coat on all sides.
2. Arrange the fillets in a wagon-wheel formation, so that 1 end of each fillet is in the center of the dish and the other end is temporarily draped over the edge of the dish.
3. Top each fillet with 1 tablespoon of onion, then fold the end of the fillet that's hanging over the edge in half over the onion.
4. When finished, you should have 4 folded-over fillets with the fold against the outer edge of the dish and the ends all in the center.
5. Cover the dish with plastic wrap, leaving a small part open at the edge to vent the steam. Microwave on high for about 3 minutes.
6. The fish is done when it just begins to separate into flakes (chunks) when pressed gently with a fork. Top the fillets with the avocado and serve them.

Nutrition:

Calories: 156

Protein: 22g

Fats: 3g

Carbohydrates: 4g

143. Tuscan Tuna and Zucchini Burgers

Preparation Time: 10 minutes

Cooking Time: 10 minutes

Servings: 2

Ingredients:

- 3 slices whole-wheat sandwich bread, toasted
- 2 (5-oz.) cans tuna in olive oil, drained
- 1 cup shredded zucchini
- 1 large egg lightly beaten

- ¼ cup diced red bell pepper
- 1 tbsp. dried oregano
- 1 tsp. lemon zest
- ¼ tsp. freshly ground black pepper
- ¼ tsp. kosher or sea salt
- 1 tbsp. extra-virgin olive oil
- Salad greens or 4 whole-wheat rolls, for serving (optional)

Directions:

1. Crumble the toast into bread crumbs using your fingers (or use a knife to cut into ¼-inch cubes) until you have 1 cup of loosely packed crumbs.
2. Pour the crumbs into a large bowl. Add the tuna, zucchini, egg bell pepper, oregano, lemon zest, black pepper and salt.
3. Mix well with a fork. With your hands, form the mixture into 4 (½ cup-size) patties. Place on a plate and press each patty flat to about ¾-inch thick.
4. In a large skillet over medium-high heat, heat the oil until it's very hot, about 2 minutes. Add the patties to the hot oil; then lower the heat to medium.
5. Cook the patties for 5 minutes. Flip with a spatula and cook for an additional 5 minutes. Enjoy as-is or serve on salad greens or whole-wheat rolls.

Nutrition:

Calories: 191

Protein: 15g

Fats: 10g

Carbohydrates: 2g

144. Sicilian Kale and Tuna Bowl

Preparation Time: 15 minutes

Cooking Time: 15 minutes

Servings: 2

Ingredients:

- 1 lb. kale
- 3 tbsps. extra-virgin olive oil
- 1 cup chopped onion

- 3 garlic cloves, minced
- 1 (2.25-oz.) can, sliced olives, drained
- ¼ cup capers
- ¼ tsp. crushed red pepper
- 2 tsps. sugar
- 2 (6-oz.) cans tuna in olive oil, undrained
- 1 (15-oz.) can cannellini beans or great northern beans
- ¼ tsp. freshly ground black pepper
- ¼ tsp. kosher or sea salt

Directions:

1. Fill a large stockpot 3-quarters full of water and bring it to a boil.
2. Add the kale and cook for 2 minutes (This is to make the kale less bitter). Drain the kale in a colander and set it aside.
3. Set the empty pot back on the stove over medium heat and pour in the oil.
4. Add the onion and cook for 4 minutes, stirring often. Add the garlic and cook for 1 minute, stirring often.
5. Add the olives, capers and crushed red pepper, and cook for 1 minute, stirring often.
6. Add the partially cooked kale and sugar, stirring until the kale is completely coated with oil.
7. Cover the pot and cook for 8 minutes.
8. Remove the kale from the heat, mix in the tuna, beans, pepper and salt, and serve.

Nutrition:

Calories: 265

Protein: 16g

Fats: 12g

Carbohydrates: 7g

145.   Mediterranean Cod Stew

Preparation Time: 10 minutes

Cooking Time: 20 minutes

Servings: 2

Ingredients:

- 2 tbsps. extra-virgin olive oil
- 2 cups chopped onion

- 2 garlic cloves, minced
- ¾ tsp. smoked paprika
- 1 (14.5-oz.) can diced tomatoes, undrained
- 1 (12-oz.) jar roasted red peppers
- 1 cup sliced olives, green or black
- 1/3 cup dry red wine
- ¼ tsp. freshly ground black pepper
- ¼ tsp. kosher or sea salt
- 1½ lbs. cod fillets, cut into 1-inch pieces
- 3 cups sliced mushrooms

Directions:

1. In a large stockpot over medium heat, heat the oil. Add the onion and cook for 4 minutes, stirring occasionally.
2. Add the garlic and smoked paprika and cook for 1 minute, stirring often.
3. Mix in the tomatoes with their juices, roasted peppers, olives, wine, pepper and salt, and turn the heat up to medium-high. Bring to a boil.
4. Add the cod and mushrooms and reduce the heat to medium.
5. Cover and cook for about 10 minutes, stirring a few times, until the cod is cooked through and flakes easily, and serve it.

Nutrition:

Calories: 220

Protein: 28g

Fats: 8g

Carbohydrates: 3g

146.   Steamed Mussels in White Wine Sauce

Preparation Time: 5 minutes

Cooking Time: 10 minutes

Servings: 2

Ingredients:

- 2 lbs. small mussels
- 1 tbsp. extra-virgin olive oil
- 1 cup thinly sliced red onion

- 3 garlic cloves, sliced
- 1 cup dry white wine
- 2 (¼-inch-thick) lemon slices
- ¼ tsp. freshly ground black pepper
- ¼ tsp. kosher or sea salt
- Fresh lemon wedges, for serving (optional)

Directions:

1. In a large colander in the sink, run cold water over the mussels (but don't let the mussels sit in standing water).
2. All the shells should be closed tight; discard any shells that are a little bit open or any shells that are cracked. Leave the mussels in the colander until you're ready to use them.
3. In a large skillet over medium-high heat, heat the oil. Add the onion and cook for 4 minutes, stirring occasionally.
4. Add the garlic and cook for 1 minute, stirring constantly. Add the wine, lemon slices, pepper and salt, and bring to a simmer. Cook for 2 minutes.
5. Add the mussels and cover. Cook for 3 minutes or until the mussels open their shells. Gently shake the pan 2 or 3 times while they are cooking.
6. All the shells should now be wide open. Using a slotted spoon, discard any mussels that are still closed. Spoon the opened mussels into a shallow serving bowl and pour the broth over the top. Serve it with additional fresh lemon slices if desired.

Nutrition:

Calories: 22

Protein: 185g

Fats: 7g

Carbohydrates: 1g

147.   Orange and Garlic Shrimp

Preparation Time: 20 minutes

Cooking Time: 10 minutes

Servings: 2

Ingredients:

- 1 large orange
- 3 tbsps. extra-virgin olive oil, divided
- 1 tbsp. chopped fresh rosemary
- 1 tbsp. chopped fresh thyme
- 3 garlic cloves, minced (about 1½ tsps.)
- ¼ tsp. freshly ground black pepper
- ¼ tsp. kosher or sea salt
- 1½ lbs. fresh raw shrimp, shells, and tails removed

Directions:

1. Zest the entire orange using a citrus grater. In a large zip-top plastic bag combine the orange zest and 2 tablespoons of oil with rosemary, thyme, garlic, pepper and salt.
2. Add the shrimp, seal the bag and gently massage the shrimp until all the ingredients are combined and the shrimp is completely covered with the seasonings. Set it aside.
3. Heat a grill, grill pan, or a large skillet over medium heat. Brush on or swirl in the remaining 1 tbsp. of oil.
4. Add half the shrimp and cook for 4 to 6 minutes, or until the shrimp turns pink and white, flipping halfway through if on the grill or stirring every minute if in a pan. Transfer the shrimp to a large serving bowl.
5. Repeat with the remaining shrimp, and add them to the bowl.
6. While the shrimp cooks, peel the orange and cut the flesh into bite-size pieces. Add to the serving bowl and toss with the cooked shrimp. Serve immediately or refrigerate and serve it cold.

Nutrition:

Calories: 190

Protein: 24g

Fats: 8g

Carbohydrates: 1g

148.   Roasted Shrimp-Gnocchi Bake

Preparation Time: 10 minutes

Cooking Time: 20 minutes

Servings: 2

Ingredients:

- 1 cup chopped fresh tomato
- 2 tbsps. extra-virgin olive oil
- 2 garlic cloves, minced
- ½ tsp. freshly ground black pepper
- ¼ tsp. crushed red pepper
- 1 (12-oz.) jar roasted red peppers
- 1 lb. fresh raw shrimp, shells and tails removed
- 1 lb. frozen gnocchi (not thawed)
- ½ cup cubed feta cheese
- 1/3 cup fresh torn basil leaves

Directions:

1. Preheat the oven to 425°F. In a baking dish, mix the tomatoes, oil, garlic, black pepper and crushed red pepper. Roast in the oven for 10 minutes.
2. Stir in the roasted peppers and shrimp. Roast for 10 more minutes, until the shrimp turns pink and white.
3. While the shrimp cooks, cook the gnocchi on the stovetop according to the package directions.
4. Drain in a colander and keep warm. Remove the dish from the oven. Mix in the cooked gnocchi, feta and basil, and serve.

Nutrition:

Calories: 227

Protein: 20g

Fats: 7g

Carbohydrates: 1g

149. Salmon Skillet Supper

Preparation Time: 15 minutes

Cooking Time: 15 minutes

Servings: 2

Ingredients:

- 1 tbsp. extra-virgin olive oil
- 2 garlic cloves minced
- 1 tsp. smoked paprika
- 1-pint grape or cherry tomatoes, quartered
- 1 (12-oz.) jar roasted red peppers
- 1 tbsp. water
- ¼ tsp. freshly ground black pepper
- ¼ tsp. kosher or sea salt
- 1 lb. salmon fillets, skin removed, cut into 8 pieces
- 1 tbsp. freshly squeezed lemon juice (from ½ medium lemon)

Directions:

1. In a large skillet over medium heat, heat the oil. Add the garlic and smoked paprika and cook for 1 minute, stirring often.
2. Add the tomatoes, roasted peppers, water, black pepper and salt. Turn up the heat to medium-high. Bring to a simmer and cook for 3 minutes, stirring occasionally and smashing the tomatoes with a wooden spoon towards the end of the cooking time.
3. Add the salmon to the skillet and spoon some of the sauce over the top.
4. Cover and cook for 10 to 12 minutes or until the salmon is cooked through (145°F using a meat thermometer) and just starts to flake.
5. Remove the skillet from the heat and drizzle lemon juice over the top of the fish. Stir the sauce, then break up the salmon into chunks with a fork. You can serve it straight from the skillet.

Nutrition:

Calories: 1168

Protein: 31g

Fats: 13g

Carbohydrates: 2g

150. Baked Cod with Vegetables

Preparation Time: 15 minutes

Cooking Time: 25 minutes

Servings: 2

Ingredients:

- 1 lb. (454g) thick cod fillet, cut into 4 even portions
- ¼ tsp. onion powder (optional)
- ¼ tsp. paprika
- 3 tbsps. extra-virgin olive oil
- 4 medium scallions
- ½ cup fresh chopped basil, divided
- 3 tbsps. minced garlic (optional)
- 2 tsps. salt
- 2 tsps. freshly ground black pepper
- ¼ tsp. dry marjoram (optional)
- 6 sun-dried tomato slices
- ½ cup dry white wine
- ½ cup crumbled feta cheese
- 1 (15-oz./425-g) can oil-packed artichoke hearts, drained
- 1 lemon, sliced
- 1 cup pitted Kalamata olives
- 1 tsp. capers (optional)
- 4 small red potatoes, quartered

Direction:

1. Set the oven to 375 °F (190 °C).
2. Season the fish with paprika and onion powder (if desired).
3. Heat an ovenproof skillet over medium heat and sear the top side of the cod for about 1 minute until golden. Set it aside.
4. Heat the olive oil in the same skillet over medium heat. Add the scallions, ¼ cup of basil, garlic (if desired), salt, pepper, marjoram (if desired), tomato slices and white wine and stir to combine. Boil; then remove it from the heat.
5. Evenly spread the sauce on the bottom of the skillet. Place the cod on top of the tomato basil sauce and scatter with feta cheese. Place the artichokes in the skillet and top with the lemon slices.
6. Scatter with the olives, capers (if desired) and the remaining ¼ cup of basil. Then, pull out from the heat and transfer it to the preheated oven. Bake it for 15 to 20 minutes
7. Meanwhile, place the quartered potatoes on a baking sheet or wrapped in aluminum foil. Bake it in the oven for 15 minutes.
8. Cool for 5 minutes before serving.

Nutrition:

Calories: 1168g

Protein: 64g

Fats: 60g

Carbohydrates: 5g

151. Slow Cooker Salmon in Foil

Preparation Time: 5 minutes

Cooking Time: 2 hours

Servings: 2

Ingredients:

- 2 (6-oz./170-g) salmon fillets
- 1 tbsp. olive oil
- 2 garlic cloves, minced
- ½ tbsp. lime juice
- 1 tsp. finely chopped fresh parsley
- ¼ tsp. black pepper

Direction

1. Spread a length of foil onto a work surface and place the salmon fillets in the middle.
2. Blend olive oil, garlic, lime juice, parsley and black pepper. Brush the mixture over the fillets. Fold the foil over and crimp the sides to make a packet.
3. Place the packet into the slow cooker. Cover and cook on High for 2 hours
4. Serve it hot.

Nutrition:

Calories: 446g

Protein: 65g

Fats: 21g

Carbohydrates: 5g

152. Dill Chutney Salmon

Preparation Time: 5 minutes

Cooking Time: 3 minutes

Servings: 2

Ingredients:

Chutney:

- ¼ cup fresh dill
- ¼ cup extra virgin olive oil
- ½ lemon juice
- Sea salt, to taste

Fish:

- 2 cups water
- 2 salmon fillets
- ½ lemon juice
- ¼ tsp. paprika
- Salt and freshly ground pepper to taste

Direction:

1. Pulse all the chutney ingredients in a food processor until creamy. Set it aside.
2. Add the water and steamer basket to the Instant Pot. Place salmon fillets, skin-side down, on the steamer basket. Drizzle the lemon juice over the salmon and sprinkle with the paprika.
3. Secure the lid. Select the Manual mode and set the cooking time for 3 minutes at High Pressure.
4. Once cooking is complete, do a quick pressure release. Carefully open the lid.
5. Season the fillets with pepper and salt to taste. Serve it topped with the dill chutney.

Nutrition:

Calories: 636g

Protein: 65g

Fats: 41g

Carbohydrates: 5g

153.   Garlic-Butter Parmesan Salmon and Asparagus

Preparation Time: 10 minutes

Cooking Time: 15 minutes

Servings: 2

Ingredients:

- 2 (6-oz./170-g) salmon fillets, skin on and patted dry
- Pink Himalayan salt
- Freshly ground black pepper, to taste
- 1 lb. (454g) fresh asparagus, ends snapped off
- 3 tbsps. almond butter
- 2 garlic cloves, minced
- ¼ cup grated Parmesan cheese

Direction:

1. Prep oven to 400 °F (205 °C). Line a baking sheet with aluminum foil.
2. Season both sides of the salmon fillets.
3. Situate the salmon in the middle of the baking sheet and arrange the asparagus around the salmon.
4. Heat the almond butter in a small saucepan over medium heat.
5. Cook the minced garlic
6. Drizzle the garlic-butter sauce over the salmon and asparagus and scatter the Parmesan cheese on top.
7. Bake in the preheated oven for about 12 minutes. You can switch the oven to broil at the end of cooking time for about 3 minutes to get a nice char on the asparagus.
8. Let cool for 5 minutes before serving.

Nutrition:

Calories: 435

Protein: 42g

Fats: 26g

Carbohydrates: 5g

154.   Lemon Rosemary Roasted Branzino

Preparation Time: 15 minutes

Cooking Time: 30 minutes

Servings: 2

Ingredients:

- 4 tbsps. extra-virgin olive oil, divided

- 2 (8-oz.) Branzino fillets
- 1 garlic clove, minced
- 1 bunch scallions
- 10 to 12 small cherry tomatoes, halved
- 1 large carrot, cut into ¼-inch rounds
- ½ cup dry white wine
- 2 tbsps. paprika
- 2 tsps. kosher salt
- ½ tbsp. ground chili pepper
- 2 rosemary sprigs or 1 tbsp. dried rosemary
- 1 small lemon, thinly sliced
- ½ cup sliced pitted Kalamata olives

Direction:

1. Heat a large ovenproof skillet over high heat until hot, about 2 minutes. Add 1 tbsp. of olive oil and heat it.
2. Add the Branzino fillets, skin-side up, and sear for 2 minutes. Flip the fillets and cook. Set them aside.
3. Swirl 2 tbsps. of olive oil around the skillet to coat evenly.
4. Add the garlic, scallions, tomatoes, and carrot, and sauté for 5 minutes.
5. Add the wine, stirring until all the ingredients are well combined. Carefully place the fish over the sauce.
6. Preheat the oven to 450 °F (235 °C).
7. Brush the fillets with the remaining 1 tablespoon of olive oil and season with paprika, salt and chili pepper. Top each fillet with a rosemary sprig and lemon slices. Scatter the olives over the fish and around the skillet.
8. Roast for about 10 minutes until the lemon slices are browned. Serve it hot.

Nutrition:

Calories: 724

Protein: 57g

Fats: 43g

Carbohydrates: 5g

155. Grilled Lemon Pesto Salmon

Preparation Time: 5 minutes

Cooking Time: 10 minutes

Servings: 2

Ingredients:

- 10 oz. (283g) salmon fillet
- 2 tbsps. prepared pesto sauce
- 1 large fresh lemon, sliced
- Cooking spray

Direction:

1. Preheat the grill to medium-high heat. Spray the grill grates with cooking spray.
2. Season the salmon well. Spread the pesto sauce on top.
3. Make a bed of fresh lemon slices about the same size as the salmon fillet on the hot grill and place the salmon on top of the lemon slices. Put any additional lemon slices on top of the salmon.
4. Grill the salmon for 10 minutes.
5. Serve it hot.

Nutrition:

Calories: 316

Protein: 29g

Fats: 21g

Carbohydrates: 5g

156. Steamed Trout with Lemon Herb Crust

Preparation Time: 10 minutes

Cooking Time: 15 minutes

Servings: 2

Ingredients:

- 3 tbsps. olive oil
- 3 garlic cloves, chopped
- 2 tbsps. fresh lemon juice
- 1 tbsp. chopped fresh mint
- 1 tbsp. chopped fresh parsley
- ¼ tsp. dried ground thyme
- 1 tsp. sea salt
- 1 lb. (454g) fresh trout (2 pieces)
- 2 cups fish stock

Direction:

1. Blend olive oil, garlic, lemon juice, mint, parsley, thyme and salt. Brush the marinade onto the fish.
2. Insert a trivet in the Instant Pot. Fill in the fish stock and place the fish on the trivet.
3. Secure the lid. Select the Steam mode and set the cooking time for 15 minutes at High Pressure.
4. Once cooking is complete, do a quick pressure release. Carefully open the lid. Serve warm.

Nutrition:

Calories: 477

Protein: 52g

Fats: 30g

Carbohydrates: 5g

157. Roasted Trout Stuffed with Veggies

Preparation Time: 10 minutes

Cooking Time: 25 minutes

Servings: 2

Ingredient:

- 2 (8-oz.) whole trout fillets
- 1 tbsp. extra-virgin olive oil
- ¼ tsp. salt
- 1/8 tsp. black pepper
- 1 small onion, thinly sliced
- ½ red bell pepper
- 1 Poblano pepper
- 2 or 3 shiitake mushrooms, sliced
- 1 lemon, sliced

Direction:

1. Set the oven to 425 °F (220 °C). Coat a baking sheet with nonstick cooking spray.
2. Rub both trout fillets, inside and out, with the olive oil. Season with salt and pepper.
3. Mix together the onion, bell pepper, Poblano pepper and mushrooms in a large bowl. Stuff half of this mix into the

cavity of each fillet. Top the mixture with 2 or 3 lemon slices inside each fillet.
4. Place the fish on the prepared baking sheet side by side. Roast in the preheated oven for 25 minutes
5. Then, pull out from the oven and serve on a plate.

Nutrition:

Calories: 453

Protein: 49g

Fats: 22g

Carbohydrates: 10g

158. Spicy Shrimp Puttanesca

Preparation Time: 5 minutes

Cooking Time: 15 minutes

Servings: 2

Ingredients:

- 2 tbsps. extra-virgin olive oil
- 3 anchovy fillets, drained and chopped
- 3 garlic cloves, minced
- ½ tsp. crushed red pepper
- 1 (14.5-oz.) can low-sodium or no-salt-added diced tomatoes, undrained
- 1 (2.25-oz.) can slice black olives, drained
- 2 tbsps. capers
- 1 tbsp. chopped fresh oregano
- 1 lb. fresh raw shrimp, shells and tails removed

Directions:

1. In a large skillet over medium heat, heat the oil. Mix in the anchovies, garlic and crushed red pepper.
2. Cook for 3 minutes, stirring frequently and mashing up the anchovies with a wooden spoon until they have melted into the oil.
3. Stir in the tomatoes with their juices, olives, capers and oregano. Turn up the heat to medium-high and bring to a simmer.
4. When the sauce is lightly bubbling, stir in the shrimp. Reduce the heat to medium

and cook the shrimp for 6 to 8 minutes, or until they turn pink and white, stirring occasionally, and serve it.

Nutrition:

Calories: 214

Protein: 26g

Fats: 10g

Carbohydrates: 2g

159. Lemony Trout with Caramelized Shallots

Preparation Time: 10 minutes

Cooking Time: 20 minutes

Servings: 2

Ingredients:

Shallots:

- 1 tsp. almond butter
- 2 shallots, thinly sliced
- Dash salt

Trout:

- 1 tbsp. almond butter
- 2 (4-oz./113-g) trout fillets
- 3 tbsps. capers
- ¼ cup freshly squeezed lemon juice
- ¼ tsp. salt
- Dash freshly grounds black pepper
- 1 lemon, thinly sliced

Direction:

For Shallots:

1. Situate the skillet over medium heat, cook the butter, shallots and salt for 20 minutes, stirring every 5 minutes.

For Trout:

2. Meanwhile, in another large skillet over medium heat, heat 1 tsp. of almond butter.
3. Add the trout fillets and cook each side for 3 minutes or until flaky. Transfer it to a plate and set them aside.

4. In the skillet used for the trout, stir in the capers, lemon juice, salt and pepper and bring to a simmer. Whisk in the remaining 1 tablespoon of almond butter. Spoon the sauce over the fish.
5. Garnish the fish with lemon slices and caramelized shallots before serving.

Nutrition:

Calories: 344

Protein: 21g

Fats: 18g

Carbohydrates: 5g

160. Easy Tomato Tuna Melts

Preparation Time: 5 minutes

Cooking Time: 4 minutes

Servings: 2

Ingredients:

- 1 (5 oz.) can chunk light tuna packed in water
- 2 tbsps. plain Greek yogurt
- 2 tbsps. finely chopped celery
- 1 tbsp. finely chopped red onion
- 2 tsps. freshly squeezed lemon juice
- 1 large tomato, cut into ¾-inch-thick rounds
- ½ cup shredded Cheddar cheese
- Cayenne pepper

Direction:

1. Preheat the broiler to high.
2. Stir together the tuna, yogurt, celery, red onion, lemon juice and cayenne pepper in a medium bowl.
3. Place the tomato rounds on a baking sheet. Top each with some tuna salad and Cheddar cheese.
4. Broil for 3 to 4 minutes until the cheese is melted and bubbly. Cool for 5 minutes before serving.

Nutrition:

Calories: 244

Protein: 30g

Fats: 10g

Carbohydrates: 7g

161.   Mackerel and Green Bean Salad

Preparation Time: 10 minutes

Cooking Time: 10 minutes

Servings: 2

Ingredients:

- 2 cups green beans
- 1 tbsp. avocado oil
- 2 mackerel fillets
- 4 cups mixed salad greens
- 2 hard-boiled eggs, sliced
- 1 avocado, sliced
- 2 tbsps. lemon juice
- 2 tbsps. olive oil
- 1 tsp. Dijon mustard
- Salt and black pepper, to taste

Direction:

1. Cook the green beans in a pot of boiling water for about 3 minutes. Drain and set aside.
2. Melt the avocado oil in a pan over medium heat. Add the mackerel fillets and cook each side for 4 minutes.
3. Divide the greens between 2 salad bowls. Top with the mackerel, sliced egg and avocado slices.
4. Scourge lemon juice, olive oil, mustard, salt and pepper, and drizzle over the salad. Add the cooked green beans and toss to combine, then serve.

Nutrition:

Calories: 737

Protein: 34g

Fats: 57g

Carbohydrates: 3g

162.   Hazelnut Crusted Sea Bass

Preparation Time: 10 minutes

Cooking Time: 15 minutes

Servings: 2

Ingredients:

- 2 tbsps. almond butter
- 2 sea bass fillets
- 1/3 cup roasted hazelnuts
- A pinch of cayenne pepper

Direction

1. Ready the oven to 425 °F (220 °C). Line a baking dish with waxed paper.
2. Brush the almond butter over the fillets.
3. Pulse the hazelnuts and cayenne in a food processor. Coat the sea bass with the hazelnut mixture, then transfer to the baking dish.
4. Bake in the preheated oven for about 15 minutes. Cool for 5 minutes before serving.

Nutrition:

Calories: 468

Protein: 40g

Fats: 31g

Carbohydrates: 5g

163.   Shrimp and Pea Paella

Preparation Time: 20 minutes

Cooking Time: 60 minutes

Servings: 2

Ingredients:

- 2 tbsps. olive oil
- 1 garlic clove, minced
- ½ large onion, minced
- 1 cup diced tomato
- ½ cup short-grain rice
- ½ tsp. sweet paprika
- ½ cup dry white wine
- 1¼ cups low-sodium chicken stock
- 8 oz. (227g) large raw shrimp
- 1 cup frozen peas
- ¼ cup jarred roasted red peppers

Direction

1. Heat the olive oil in a large skillet over medium-high heat.
2. Add the garlic and onion and sauté for 3 minutes or until the onion is softened.
3. Add the tomato, rice and paprika and stir for 3 minutes to toast the rice.
4. Add the wine and chicken stock and stir to combine. Bring the mixture to a boil.
5. Cover and set the heat to medium-low and simmer for 45 minutes
6. Add the shrimp, peas and roasted red peppers. Cover and cook for an additional 5 minutes. Season with salt to taste and serve.

Nutrition:

Calories: 646

Protein: 42g

Fats: 27g

Carbohydrates: 1g

164.   Garlic Shrimp with Arugula Pesto

Preparation Time: 20 minutes

Cooking Time: 5 minutes

Servings: 2

Ingredients:

- 3 cups lightly packed arugula
- ½ cup lightly packed basil leaves
- ¼ cup walnuts
- 3 tbsps. olive oil
- 3 medium garlic cloves
- 2 tbsps. grated Parmesan cheese
- 1 tbsp. freshly squeezed lemon juice
- 1 (10-oz.) package zucchini noodles
- 8 oz. (227g) cooked, shelled shrimp
- 2 Roma tomatoes, diced

Direction

1. Process the arugula, basil, walnuts, olive oil, garlic, Parmesan cheese and lemon juice in a food processor until smooth, scraping down the sides as needed. Season

2. Heat a skillet over medium heat. Add the pesto, zucchini noodles and cooked shrimp. Toss to combine the sauce over the noodles and shrimp and cook until heated through.
3. Season well. Serve topped with the diced tomatoes.

Nutrition:

Calories: 435

Protein: 33g

Fats: 30.2g

Carbohydrates: 8g

165.   Baked Oysters with Vegetables

Preparation Time: 30 minutes

Cooking Time: 17 minutes

Servings: 2

Ingredients:

- 2 cups coarse salt, for holding the oysters
- 1 dozen fresh oysters, scrubbed
- 1 tbsp., almond butter
- ¼ cup finely chopped scallions
- ½ cup finely chopped artichoke hearts
- ¼ cup finely chopped red bell pepper
- 1 garlic clove, minced
- 1 tbsp. finely chopped fresh parsley
- Zest and juice of ½ lemon

Direction:

1. Pour the salt into a baking dish and spread to fill the bottom of the dish evenly.
2. Using a shucking knife, insert the blade at the joint of the shell, where it hinges open and shut. Firmly apply pressure to pop the blade in and work the knife around the shell to open. Discard the empty half of the shell. Using the knife, gently loosen the oyster, and remove any shell particles. Sprinkle salt in the oysters.
3. Set the oven to 425 °F (220 °C).
4. Heat the almond butter in a large skillet over medium heat. Add the scallions,

artichoke hearts and bell pepper, and cook for 5 to 7 minutes. Cook the garlic.

5. Retire from the heat and stir in the parsley, lemon zest and juice, and season to taste with salt and pepper.
6. Divide the vegetable mixture evenly among the oysters. Bake in the preheated oven for 10 to 12 minutes.

Nutrition:

Calories: 35

Protein: 6g

Fats: 7g

Carbohydrates: 4g

166.   Creamy Fish Gratin

Preparation Time: 10 minutes

Cooking Time: 55 minutes

Servings: 2

Ingredients:

-   1/3 cup heavy cream
-   1 cubed salmon fillet
-   1 cod fillet, cubed
-   1 sea bass fillet, cubed
-   1/3 celery stalk, sliced
-   Salt and pepper
-   1/3 cup grated Parmesan
-   1/3 cup crumbled feta cheese

Directions:

1. Combine the cream with the fish fillets and celery in a deep-dish baking pan.
2. Add salt and pepper to taste, then top with the Parmesan and feta cheese.
3. Cook in the preheated oven at 350°F/176°C for 20 minutes.
4. Serve the gratin and enjoy it.

Nutrition:

Calories: 301

Protein: 36.9g

Fats: 16.1g

Carbohydrates: 1.3g

167.   Mixed Seafood Dish

Preparation Time: 10 minutes

Cooking Time: 35 minutes

Servings: 2

Ingredients:

-   6 scrubbed clams, cleaned
-   2 chopped dried chilies, soaked and drained
-   ½ lobster, tail separated and halved
-   ½ cup water
-   1/8 cup flour
-   2 tbsps. olive oil
-   1 lb. or 500g skinless monkfish, boneless and thinly sliced into fillets
-   Salt and black pepper
-   18 unpeeled shrimp
-   ½ chopped onion
-   2 minced garlic cloves
-   2 grated tomatoes
-   ½ baguette slice, toasted
-   15 skinned hazelnuts
-   1 tbsp. chopped parsley
-   ½ cup fish stock
-   1/8 tsp. smoked paprika
-   Lemon wedges
-   Crusty bread slices

Directions:

1. Put the water in a large saucepan and bring to a boil over high heat.
2. Add the clams, cover and cook for 4 minutes. Take it away from the heat and discard the unopened ones.
3. Heat a skillet with olive oil over medium-high heat.
4. In the meantime, put flour on a medium bowl and dredge in the fish.
5. Season with salt and pepper.
6. Place the fish into the skillet and cook for 3 minutes on each side, after transfer it to a plate.
7. Add the shrimps to the same skillet and cook for about 2 minutes on each side. Transfer them to a plate.

8. Reduce the heat to medium-low, add the garlic to the same pan. Stir; cook for 1 minute and transfer to a blender.
9. Add the onion to the skillet and stir for 3 minutes.
10. Add the tomatoes. Stir and cook on low heat for 7 minutes.

Nutrition:

Calories: 344

Protein: 21g

Fats: 18g

Carbohydrates: 5g

Bean, Pasta and Rice Recipes

168. Rice with Vermicelli

Preparation Time: 5 minutes

Cooking Time: 45 minutes

Servings: 6

Ingredients:

- 2 cups short-grain rice
- 3½ cups water, plus more for rinsing and soaking the rice
- ¼ cup olive oil
- 1 cup broken vermicelli pasta
- Salt

Directions:

1. Soak the rice under cold water until the water runs clean. Place the rice in a bowl, cover with water, and let soak for 10 minutes. Drain and set aside. Cook the olive oil in a medium pot over medium heat.
2. Stir in the vermicelli and cook for 2 to 3 minutes, stirring continuously, until golden.
3. Put the rice and cook for 1 minute, stirring, so the rice is well coated in the oil. Stir in the water and a pinch of salt and bring the liquid to a boil. Adjust heat and simmer for 20 minutes. Pull out from the heat and let rest for 10 minutes. Fluff with a fork and serve.

Nutrition (for 100g):

346 calories

9g total fat

60g carbohydrates

2g protein

0.9mg sodium

169. Fava Beans and Rice

Preparation Time: 10 minutes

Cooking Time: 35 minutes

Servings: 4

Difficulty Level: Easy

Ingredients:

- ¼ cup olive oil
- 4 cups fresh fava beans, shelled
- 4½ cups water, plus more for drizzling
- 2 cups basmati rice
- 1/8 teaspoon salt
- 1/8 teaspoon freshly ground black pepper
- 2 tablespoons pine nuts, toasted
- ½ cup chopped fresh garlic chives, or fresh onion chives

Directions:

1. Fill the sauce pan with olive oil and cook over medium heat. Add the fava beans and drizzle them with a bit of water to avoid burning or sticking. Cook for 10 minutes.
2. Gently stir in the rice. Add the water, salt, and pepper. Set up the heat and boil the mixture. Adjust the heat and let it simmer for 15 minutes.
3. Pull out from the heat and let it rest for 10 minutes before serving. Spoon onto a serving platter and sprinkle with the toasted pine nuts and chives.

Nutrition (for 100g):

587 calories

17g total fat

97g carbohydrates

2g protein

0.6mg sodium

170. Buttered Fava Beans

Preparation Time: 30 minutes

Cooking Time: 15 minutes

Servings: 4

Difficulty Level: Easy

Ingredients:

- ½ cup vegetable broth
- 4 pounds fava beans, shelled
- ¼ cup fresh tarragon, divided
- 1 teaspoon chopped fresh thyme
- ¼ teaspoon freshly ground black pepper
- 1/8 teaspoon salt
- 2 tablespoons butter
- 1 garlic clove, minced
- 2 tablespoons chopped fresh parsley

Directions:

1. Boil vegetable broth in a shallow pan over medium heat. Add the fava beans, 2 tablespoons of tarragon, the thyme, pepper, and salt. Cook until the broth is almost absorbed and the beans are tender.
2. Stir in the butter, garlic, and remaining 2 tablespoons of tarragon. Cook for 2 to 3 minutes. Sprinkle with the parsley and serve hot.

Nutrition (for 100g):

458 calories

9g fat

81g carbohydrates

37g protein

691mg sodium

171. Freekeh

Preparation Time: 10 minutes

Cooking Time: 40 minutes

Servings: 4

Difficulty Level: Easy

Ingredients:

- 4 tablespoons Ghee
- 1 onion, chopped
- 3½ cups vegetable broth
- 1 teaspoon ground allspice
- 2 cups freekeh
- 2 tablespoons pine nuts, toasted

Directions:

1. Melt ghee in a heavy-bottomed saucepan over medium heat. Stir in the onion and cook for about 5 minutes, stirring constantly, until the onion is golden. Pour in the vegetable broth, add the allspice, and bring to a boil. Stir in the freekeh and return the mixture to a boil. Adjust heat and simmer for 30 minutes, stir occasionally. Spoon the freekeh into a serving dish and top with the toasted pine nuts.

Nutrition (for 100g):

459 calories

18g fat

64g carbohydrates

10g protein

692mg sodium

172. Fried Rice Balls with Tomato Sauce

Preparation Time: 15 minutes

Cooking Time: 20 minutes

Servings: 8

Ingredients:

- 1 cup bread crumbs
- 2 cups cooked risotto
- 2 large eggs, divided
- ¼ cup freshly grated Parmesan cheese
- 8 fresh baby mozzarella balls, or 1 (4-inch) log fresh mozzarella, cut into 8 pieces
- 2 tablespoons water
- 1 cup corn oil
- 1 cup Basic Tomato Basil Sauce, or store-bought

Directions:

2. Situate the bread crumbs into a small bowl and set aside. In a medium bowl, stir together the risotto, 1 egg, and the Parmesan cheese until well combined. Split the risotto mixture into 8 pieces.

Situate them on a clean work surface and flatten each piece.

3. Place 1 mozzarella ball on each flattened rice disk. Close the rice around the mozzarella to form a ball. Repeat until you finish all the balls. In the same medium, now-empty bowl, whisk the remaining egg and the water. Dip each prepared risotto ball into the egg wash and roll it in the bread crumbs. Set aside.

4. Cook corn oil in a skillet over high heat. Gently lower the risotto balls into the hot oil and fry for 5 to 8 minutes until golden brown. Stir them, as needed, to ensure the entire surface is fried. Using a slotted spoon, put the fried balls to paper towels to drain.

5. Warm up the tomato sauce in a medium saucepan over medium heat for 5 minutes, stir occasionally, and serve the warm sauce alongside the rice balls.

Nutrition (for 100g):

255 calories

15g fat

16g carbohydrates

2g protein

669mg sodium

173.   Spanish-Style Rice

Preparation Time: 10 minutes

Cooking Time: 35 minutes

Servings: 4

Difficulty Level: Average

Ingredients:

- ¼ cup olive oil
- 1 small onion, finely chopped
- 1 red bell pepper, seeded and diced
- 1½ cups white rice
- 1 teaspoon sweet paprika
- ½ teaspoon ground cumin
- ½ teaspoon ground coriander
- 1 garlic clove, minced

- 3 tablespoons tomato paste
- 3 cups vegetable broth
- 1/8 teaspoon salt

Directions:

1. Cook the olive oil in a large heavy-bottomed skillet over medium heat. Stir in the onion and red bell pepper. Cook for 5 minutes or until softened. Add the rice, paprika, cumin, and coriander and cook for 2 minutes, stirring often.

2. Add the garlic, tomato paste, vegetable broth, and salt. Stir it well and season, as needed. Allow the mixture to a boil. Lower heat and simmer for 20 minutes.

3. Set aside for 5 minutes before serving.

Nutrition (for 100g):

414 calories

14g fat

63g carbohydrates

2g protein

664mg sodium

174.   Zucchini with Rice and Tzatziki

Preparation Time: 20 minutes

Cooking Time: 35 minutes

Servings: 4

Ingredients:

- ¼ cup olive oil
- 1 onion, chopped
- 3 zucchinis, diced
- 1 cup vegetable broth
- ½ cup chopped fresh dill
- Salt
- Freshly ground black pepper
- 1 cup short-grain rice
- 2 tablespoons pine nuts
- 1 cup Tzatziki Sauce, Plain Yogurt, or store-bought

Directions:

1. Cook oil in a heavy-bottomed pot over medium heat. Stir in the onion, turn the heat to medium-low, and sauté for 5 minutes. Mix in the zucchini and cook for 2 minutes more.
2. Stir in the vegetable broth and dill and season with salt and pepper. Turn up heat to medium and bring the mixture to a boil.
3. Stir in the rice and place the mixture back to a boil. Set the heat to very low, cover the pot, and cook for 15 minutes. Pull out from the heat and set aside, for 10 minutes. Scoop the rice onto a serving platter, sprinkle with the pine nuts, and serve with tzatziki sauce.

Nutrition (for 100g):

414 calories

17g fat

57g carbohydrates

5g protein

591mg sodium

175.   Cannellini Beans with Rosemary and Garlic Aioli

Preparation Time: 10 minutes

Cooking Time: 10 minutes

Servings: 4

Ingredients:

- 4 cups cooked cannellini beans
- 4 cups water
- ½ teaspoon salt
- 3 tablespoons olive oil
- 2 tablespoons chopped fresh rosemary
- ½ cup Garlic Aioli
- ¼ teaspoon freshly ground black pepper

Directions:

1. Mix the cannellini beans, water, and salt in a medium saucepan over medium heat. Bring to a boil. Cook for 5 minutes. Drain. Cook the olive oil in a skillet over medium heat.

2. Add the beans. Stir in the rosemary and aioli. Adjust heat to medium-low and cook, stirring, just to heat through. Season with pepper and serve.

Nutrition (for 100g):

545 calories

36g fat

42g carbohydrates

14g protein

608mg sodium

176.   Jeweled Rice

Preparation Time: 15 minutes

Cooking Time: 30 minutes

Servings: 6

Ingredients:

- ½ cup olive oil, divided
- 1 onion, finely chopped
- 1 garlic clove, minced
- ½ teaspoon chopped peeled fresh ginger
- 4½ cups water
- 1 teaspoon salt, divided, plus more as needed
- 1 teaspoon ground turmeric
- 2 cups basmati rice
- 1 cup fresh sweet peas
- 2 carrots, peeled and cut into ½-inch dice
- ½ cup dried cranberries
- Grated zest of 1 orange
- 1/8 teaspoon cayenne pepper
- ¼ cup slivered almonds, toasted

Directions:

1. Warm up ¼ cup of olive oil in a large pan. Place the onion and cook for 4 minutes. Sauté in the garlic and ginger.
2. Stir in the water, ¾ teaspoon of salt, and the turmeric. Bring the mixture to a boil. Put in the rice and return the mixture to a boil. Taste the broth and season with more salt, as needed. Select the heat to low, and cook for 15 minutes. Turn off

the heat. Let the rice rest on the burner, covered, for 10 minutes. Meanwhile, in a medium sauté pan or skillet over medium-low heat, heat the remaining ¼ cup of olive oil. Stir in the peas and carrots. Cook for 5 minutes.

3. Stir in the cranberries and orange zest. Dust with the remaining salt and the cayenne. Cook for 1 to 2 minutes. Spoon the rice onto a serving platter. Top with the peas and carrots and sprinkle with the toasted almonds.

Nutrition (for 100g):

460 calories

19g fat

65g carbohydrates

4g protein

810mg sodium

177.   Asparagus Risotto

Preparation Time: 15 minutes

Cooking Time: 30 minutes

Servings: 4

Ingredients:

- 5 cups vegetable broth, divided
- 3 tablespoons unsalted butter, divided
- 1 tablespoon olive oil
- 1 small onion, chopped
- 1½ cups Arborio rice
- 1-pound fresh asparagus, ends trimmed, cut into 1-inch pieces, tips separated
- ¼ cup freshly grated Parmesan cheese

Directions:

1. Boil the vegetable broth over medium heat. Set the heat to low and simmer. Mix 2 tablespoons of butter with the olive oil. Stir in the onion and cook for 2 to 3 minutes.
2. Put the rice and stir with a wooden spoon while cooking for 1 minute until the grains are well covered with butter and oil.

3. Stir in ½ cup of warm broth. Cook and continue stirring until the broth is completely absorbed. Add the asparagus stalks and another ½ cup of broth. Cook and stir occasionally Continue adding the broth, ½ cup at a time, and cooking until it is completely absorbed upon adding the next ½ cup. Stir frequently to prevent sticking. Rice should be cooked but still firm.
4. Add the asparagus tips, the remaining 1 tablespoon of butter, and the Parmesan cheese. Stir vigorously to combine. Remove from the heat, top with additional Parmesan cheese, if desired, and serve immediately.

Nutrition (for 100g):

434 calories

14g fat

67g carbohydrates

6g protein

517mg sodium

178.   Vegetable Paella

Preparation Time: 25 minutes

Cooking Time: 45 minutes

Servings: 6

Ingredients:

- ¼ cup olive oil
- 1 large sweet onion
- 1 large red bell pepper
- 1 large green bell pepper
- 3 garlic cloves, finely minced
- 1 teaspoon smoked paprika
- 5 saffron threads
- 1 zucchini, cut into ½-inch cubes
- 4 large ripe tomatoes, peeled, seeded, and chopped
- 1½ cups short-grain Spanish rice
- 3 cups vegetable broth, warmed

Directions:

1. Preheat the oven to 350°F. Cook the olive oil over medium heat. Stir in the onion and red and green bell peppers and cook for 10 minutes.
2. Stir in the garlic, paprika, saffron threads, zucchini, and tomatoes. Turn down the heat to medium-low and cook for 10 minutes.
3. Stir in the rice and vegetable broth. Increase the heat to bring the paella to a boil. Put the heat to medium-low and cook for 15 minutes. Wrap the pan with aluminum foil and put it in the oven.
4. Bake for 10 minutes or until the broth is absorbed.

Nutrition (for 100g):

288 calories

10g fat

46g carbohydrates

3g protein

671mg sodium

179. Eggplant and Rice Casserole

Preparation Time: 30 minutes

Cooking Time: 35 minutes

Servings: 4

Ingredients:

For the Sauce

- ½ cup olive oil
- 1 small onion, chopped
- 4 garlic cloves, mashed
- 6 ripe tomatoes, peeled and chopped
- 2 tablespoons tomato paste
- 1 teaspoon dried oregano
- ¼ teaspoon ground nutmeg
- ¼ teaspoon ground cumin
- For the Casserole
- 4 (6-inch) Japanese eggplants, halved lengthwise
- 2 tablespoons olive oil
- 1 cup cooked rice
- 2 tablespoons pine nuts, toasted

- 1 cup water

Directions:

1. To Make the Sauce
2. Cook the olive oil in a heavy-bottomed saucepan over medium heat. Place the onion and cook for 5 minutes. Stir in the garlic, tomatoes, tomato paste, oregano, nutmeg, and cumin. Boil then down heat to low, and simmer for 10 minutes. Remove and set aside.
3. To Make the Casserole
4. Preheat the broiler. While the sauce simmers, drizzle the eggplant with the olive oil and place them on a baking sheet. Broil for about 5 minutes until golden. Remove and let cool. Turn the oven to 375°F. Arrange the cooled eggplant, cut-side up, in a 9-by-13-inch baking dish. Gently scoop out some flesh to make room for the stuffing.
5. In a bowl, combine half the tomato sauce, the cooked rice, and pine nuts. Fill each eggplant half with the rice mixture. In the same bowl, combine the remaining tomato sauce and water. Pour over the eggplant. Bake, covered, for 20 minutes until the eggplant is soft.

Nutrition (for 100g):

453 calories

39g fat

29g carbohydrates

7g protein

820mg sodium

180. Many Vegetable Couscous

Preparation Time: 15 minutes

Cooking Time: 45 minutes

Servings: 8

Ingredients:

- ¼ cup olive oil
- 1 onion, chopped
- 4 garlic cloves, minced

- 2 jalapeño peppers, pierced with a fork in several places
- ½ teaspoon ground cumin
- ½ teaspoon ground coriander
- 1 (28-ounce) can crushed tomatoes
- 2 tablespoons tomato paste
- 1/8 teaspoon salt
- 2 bay leaves
- 11 cups water, divided
- 4 carrots
- 2 zucchinis, cut into 2-inch pieces
- 1 acorn squash, halved, seeded, and cut into 1-inch-thick slices
- 1 (15-ounce) can chickpeas, drained and rinsed
- ¼ cup chopped Preserved Lemons (optional)
- 3 cups couscous

Directions:

1. Cook the olive oil in heavy-bottom pot. Place the onion and cook for 4 minutes. Stir in the garlic, jalapeños, cumin, and coriander. Cook for 1 minute. Add the tomatoes, tomato paste, salt, bay leaves, and 8 cups of water. Bring the mixture to a boil.
2. Add the carrots, zucchini, and acorn squash and return to a boil. Reduce the heat slightly, cover, and cook for about 20 minutes until the vegetables are tender but not mushy. Get 2 cups of the cooking liquid and set aside. Season as needed.
3. Add the chickpeas and preserved lemons (if using). Cook for few minutes, and turn off the heat.
4. In a medium pan, bring the remaining 3 cups of water to a boil over high heat. Stir in the couscous, cover, and turn off the heat. Let the couscous rest for 10 minutes. Drizzle with 1 cup of reserved cooking liquid. Using a fork, fluff the couscous.
5. Mound it on a large platter. Drizzle it with the remaining cooking liquid. Pull out the vegetables from the pot and arrange on top. Serve the remaining stew in a separate bowl.

Nutrition (for 100g):

415 calories

7g fat

75g carbohydrates

9g protein

718mg sodium

181.   Kushari

Preparation Time: 25 minutes

Cooking Time: 1 hour and 20 minutes

Servings: 8

Ingredients:

- For the sauce
- 2 tablespoons olive oil
- 2 garlic cloves, minced
- 1 (16-ounce) can tomato sauce
- ¼ cup white vinegar
- ¼ cup Harissa, or store-bought
- 1/8 teaspoon salt
- For the rice
- 1 cup olive oil
- 2 onions, thinly sliced
- 2 cups dried brown lentils
- 4 quarts plus ½ cup water, divided
- 2 cups short-grain rice
- 1 teaspoon salt
- 1-pound short elbow pasta
- 1 (15-ounce) can chickpeas, drained and rinsed

Directions:

1. To make the sauce
2. In a saucepan, cook the olive oil. Sauté the garlic. Stir in the tomato sauce, vinegar, harissa, and salt. Bring the sauce to boil. Turn down the heat to low and cook for 20 minutes or until the sauce has thickened. Remove and set aside.
3. To make the rice
4. Ready the plate with paper towels and set aside. In a large pan over medium heat, heat the olive oil. Sauté the onions, stir often, until crisp and golden. Transfer the onions to the prepared plate and set aside.

Reserve 2 tablespoons of the cooking oil. Reserve the pan.

5. Over high heat, combine the lentils and 4 cups of water in a pot. Allow it boil and cook for 20 minutes. Strain and toss with the reserved 2 tablespoons of cooking oil. Set aside. Reserve the pot.

6. Place the pan you used to fry the onions over medium-high heat and add the rice, 4½ cups of water, and the salt to it. Bring to a boil. Set the heat to low, and cook for 20 minutes. Turn off and set aside for 10 minutes. Bring the remaining 8 cups of water, salted, to a boil over high heat in the same pot used to cook the lentils. Drop in the pasta and cook for 6 minutes or according to the package instructions. Drain and set aside.

7. To assemble

8. Spoon the rice onto a serving platter. Top it with the lentils, chickpeas, and pasta. Drizzle with the hot tomato sauce and sprinkle with the crispy fried onions.

Nutrition (for 100g):

668 calories

13g fat

113g carbohydrates

18g protein

481mg sodium

182. Bulgur with Tomatoes and Chickpeas

Preparation Time: 10 minutes

Cooking Time: 35 minutes

Servings: 6

Ingredients:

- ½ cup olive oil
- 1 onion, chopped
- 6 tomatoes, diced, or 1 (16-ounce) can diced tomatoes
- 2 tablespoons tomato paste
- 2 cups water
- 1 tablespoon Harissa, or store-bought

- 1/8 teaspoon salt
- 2 cups coarse bulgur
- 1 (15-ounce) can chickpeas, drained and rinsed

Directions:

1. In a heavy-bottomed pot over medium heat, heat up the olive oil. Sauté the onion then add the tomatoes with their juice and cook for 5 minutes.

2. Stir in the tomato paste, water, harissa, and salt. Bring to a boil.

3. Stir in the bulgur and chickpeas. Return the mixture to a boil. Decrease the heat to low and cook for 15 minutes. Let rest for 15 minutes before serving.

Nutrition (for 100g):

413 calories

19g fat

55g carbohydrates

14g protein

728mg sodium

183. Mackerel Maccheroni

Preparation Time: 10 minutes

Cooking Time: 15 minutes

Servings: 4

Ingredients

- 12oz Maccheroni
- 1 clove garlic
- 14oz Tomato sauce
- 1 sprig chopped parsley
- 2 Fresh chili peppers
- 1 teaspoon salt
- 7oz mackerel in oil
- 3 tablespoons extra virgin olive oil

Directions

1. Start by putting the water to boil in a saucepan. While the water is heating up, take a pan, pour in a little oil and a little

garlic and cook over low heat. Once the garlic is cooked, pull it out from the pan.

2. Cut open the chili pepper, remove the internal seeds and cut into thin strips.
3. Add the cooking water and the chili pepper to the same pan as before. Then, take the mackerel, and after draining the oil and separating it with a fork, put it to the pan with the other ingredients. Lightly sauté it by adding some cooking water.
4. When all the ingredients are well incorporated, add the tomato puree in the pan. Mix well to even out all the ingredients and then, cook on low heat for about 3 minutes.
5. Let's move on to the pasta:
6. After the water starts boiling, add the salt and the pasta. Drain the maccheroni once they are slightly al dente, and add them to the sauce you prepared.
7. Sauté for a few moments in the sauce and after tasting, season with salt and pepper according to your liking.

Nutrition (for 100g):

510 Calories

15.4g Fat

70g Carbohydrates

22.9g Protein

730mg Sodium

184. Maccheroni With Cherry Tomatoes and Anchovies

Preparation Time: 10 minutes

Cooking Time: 15 minutes

Servings: 4

Ingredients

- 14oz Maccheroni Pasta
- 6 Salted anchovies
- 4oz Cherry tomatoes
- 1 clove garlic
- 3 tablespoons extra virgin olive oil
- Fresh chili peppers to taste
- 3 basil leaves

- Salt to taste

Directions

1. Start by heating water in a pot and add salt when it is boiling. Meanwhile, prepare the sauce: Take the tomatoes after having washed them and cut them into 4 pieces.
2. Now, take a non-stick pan, sprinkle in a little oil and throw in a clove of garlic. Once cooked, remove it from the pan. Add the clean anchovies to the pan, melting them in the oil.
3. When the anchovies are well dissolved, add the cut tomatoes pieces and turn the heat up to high, until they begin to soften (be careful not to let them become too soft).
4. Add the chili peppers without seeds, cut into small pieces, and season.
5. Transfer the pasta in the pot of boiling water, drain it al dente, and let it sauté in the saucepan for a few moments.

Nutrition (for 100g):

476 Calories

11g Fat

81.4g Carbohydrates

12.9g Protein

763mg Sodium

185. Lemon and Shrimp Risotto

Preparation Time: 10 minutes

Cooking Time: 30 minutes

Servings: 4

Ingredients

- 1 lemon
- 14oz Shelled shrimp
- 1 ¾ cups risotto Rice
- 1 white onion
- 33 fl. oz (1 liter) vegetable broth (even less is fine)
- 2 ½ tablespoons butter
- ½ glass white wine
- Salt to taste

- Black pepper to taste
- Chives to taste

Directions

1. Start by boiling the shrimps in salted water for 3-4 minutes, drain and set aside.
2. Peel and finely chop an onion, stir fry it with melted butter and once the butter has dried, toast the rice in the pan for a few minutes.
3. Deglaze the rice with half a glass of white wine, then add the juice of 1 lemon. Stir and finish cooking the rice by continuing to add a ladle of vegetable stock as needed.
4. Mix well and a few minutes before the end of cooking, add the previously cooked shrimps (keeping some of them aside for garnish) and some black pepper.
5. Once the heat is off, add a knob of butter and stir. The risotto is ready to be served. Decorate with the remaining shrimp and sprinkle with some chives.

Nutrition (for 100g):

510 Calories

10g Fat

82.4g Carbohydrates

20.6g Protein

875mg Sodium

186.   Spaghetti with Clams

Preparation Time: 10 minutes

Cooking Time: 40 minutes

Servings: 4

Ingredients

- 11.5oz of spaghetti
- 2 pounds of clams
- 7oz of tomato sauce, or tomato pulp, for the red version of this dish
- 2 cloves of garlic
- 4 tablespoons extra virgin olive oil
- 1 glass of dry white wine
- 1 tablespoon of finely chopped parsley

- 1 chili pepper

Directions

1. Start by washing the clams: never "purge" the clams — they must only be opened through the use of heat, otherwise their precious internal liquid is lost along with any sand. Wash the clams quickly using a colander placed in a salad bowl: this will filter out the sand on the shells.
2. Then immediately put the drained clams in a saucepan with a lid on high heat. Turn them over occasionally, and when they are almost all open take them off the heat. The clams that remain closed are dead and must be eliminated. Remove the mollusks from the open ones, leaving some of them whole to decorate the dishes. Strain the liquid left at the bottom of the pan, and set aside.
3. Take a large pan and pour a little oil in it. Heat a whole pepper and one or two cloves of crushed garlic on very low heat until the cloves become yellowish. Add the clams and season with dry white wine.
4. Now, add the clam liquid strained previously and a some finely chopped parsley.
5. Strain and immediately toss the spaghetti al dente in the pan, after having cooked them in plenty of salted water. Stir well until the spaghetti absorb all the liquid from the clams. If you did not use a chili pepper, complete with a light sprinkle of white or black pepper.

Nutrition (for 100g):

167 Calories

8g Fat

18.63g Carbohydrates

5g Protein

720mg Sodium

187.   Greek Fish Soup

Preparation Time: 10 minutes

Cooking Time: 60 minutes

Servings: 4

Ingredients

- Hake or other white fish
- 4 Potatoes
- 4 Spring onions
- 2 Carrots
- 2 stalks of Celery
- 2 Tomatoes
- 4 tablespoons Extra virgin olive oil
- 2 Eggs
- 1 Lemon
- 1 cup Rice
- Salt to taste

Directions

1. Choose a fish not exceeding 2.2pounds in weight, remove its scales, gills and intestines and wash it well. Salt it and set aside.
2. Wash the potatoes, carrots and onions and put them in the saucepan whole with enough water to soak them and then bring to a boil.
3. Add in the celery still tied in bunches so it does not disperse while cooking, cut the tomatoes into four parts and add these too, together with oil and salt.
4. When the vegetables are almost cooked, add more water and the fish. Boil for 20 minutes then remove it from the broth together with the vegetables.
5. Place the fish in a serving dish by adorning it with the vegetables and strain the broth. Put the broth back on the heat, diluting it with a little water. Once it boils, put in the rice and season with salt. Once the rice is cooked, remove the saucepan from the heat.
6. Prepare the avgolemono sauce:
7. Beat the eggs well and slowly add the lemon juice. Put some broth in a ladle and slowly pour it into the eggs, mixing constantly.
8. Finally, add the obtained sauce to the soup and mix well.

Nutrition (for 100g):

263 Calories

17.1g Fat

18.6g Carbohydrates

9g Protein

823mg Sodium

188.   Venere Rice with Shrimp

Preparation Time: 10 minutes

Cooking Time: 55 minutes

Servings: 3

Ingredients

- 1 ½ cups of black Venere rice (better if parboiled)
- 5 teaspoons extra virgin olive oil
- 10.5oz shrimp
- 10.5oz zucchini
- 1 Lemon (juice and rind)
- Table Salt to taste
- Black pepper to taste
- 1 clove garlic
- Tabasco to taste

Directions

1. Let's start with the rice:
2. After filling a pot with plenty of water and bringing it to a boil, pour in the rice, add salt and cook for the necessary time (check the cooking instructions on the package).
3. Meanwhile, grate the zucchini with grater with large holes. In a pan, heat up the olive oil with the peeled garlic clove, add the grated zucchini, salt and pepper, and cook for 5 minutes, then, remove the garlic clove and set the vegetables aside.
4. Now clean the shrimp:
5. Remove the shell, cut the tail and divide them in half lengthwise, remove the intestine (the dark thread in their back). Situate the cleaned shrimps in a bowl and season with olive oil; give it some extra flavor by adding lemon zest, salt and pepper and by adding a few drops of Tabasco if you so choose.

6. Heat up the shrimps in a hot pan for a couple of minutes. Once cooked, set aside.
7. Once the Venere rice is ready, strain it in a bowl, add the zucchini mix and stir.

Nutrition (for 100g):

293 Calories

5g Fat

52g Carbohydrates

10g Protein

655mg Sodium

189. Pennette with Salmon and Vodka

Preparation Time: 10 minutes

Cooking Time: 18 minutes

Servings: 4

Ingredients

- 14oz Pennette Rigate
- 7oz Smoked salmon
- 1.2oz Shallot
  o fl. oz(40ml) Vodka
- 5 oz cherry tomatoes
- 7 oz fresh liquid cream (I recommend the vegetable one for a lighter dish)
- Chives to taste
- 3 tablespoons extra virgin olive oil
- Salt to taste
- Black pepper to taste
- Basil to taste (for garnish)

Directions

2. Wash and cut the tomatoes and the chives. After having peeled the shallot, chop it with a knife, put it in a saucepan and let it marinate in extra virgin olive oil for a few moments.
3. Meanwhile, cut the salmon into strips and sauté it together with the oil and shallot.
4. Blend everything with the vodka, being careful as there could be a flare (if a flame should rise, don't worry, it will lower as soon as the alcohol has evaporated

completely). Add the chopped tomatoes and add a pinch of salt and, if you like, some pepper. Finally, add the cream and chopped chives.
5. While the sauce continues cooking, prepare the pasta. Once the water boils, pour in the Pennette and let them cook until al dente.
6. Strain the pasta, and pour the Pennette into the sauce, letting them cook for a few moments so as allow them to absorb all the flavor. If you like, garnish with a basil leaf.

Nutrition (for 100g):

620 Calories

21.9g Fat

81.7g Carbohydrates

24g Protein

326mg Sodium

190. Seafood Carbonara

Preparation Time: 15 minutes

Cooking Time: 50 minutes

Servings: 3

Ingredients

- 11.5oz Spaghetti
- 3.5oz Tuna
- 3.5oz Swordfish
- 3.5oz Salmon
- 6 Yolks
- 4 tablespoons Parmesan cheese (Parmigiano Reggiano)
- 2 fl. oz (60ml) White wine
- 1 clove garlic
- Extra virgin olive oil to taste
- Table Salt to taste
- Black pepper to taste

Directions

1. Prepare a boiling water in a pot and add a little salt.

2. Meanwhile, pour 6 egg yolks in a bowl and add the grated parmesan, pepper and salt. Beat with a whisk, and dilute with a little cooking water from the pot.
3. Remove any bones from the salmon, the scales from the swordfish, and proceed by dicing the tuna, salmon and swordfish.
4. Once it boils, toss in the pasta and cook it slightly al dente.
5. Meanwhile, heat a little oil in a large pan, add the whole peeled garlic clove. Once the oil is hot, toss in the fish cubes and sauté over high heat for about 1 minute. Remove the garlic and add the white wine.
6. Once the alcohol evaporates, take out the fish cubes and lower the heat. As soon as the spaghetti are ready, add them to the pan and sauté for about a minute, stirring constantly and adding the cooking water, as needed.
7. Pour in the egg yolk mixture and the fish cubes. Mix well. Serve.

Nutrition (for 100g):

375 Calories

17g Fat

41.40g Carbohydrates

14g Protein

755 mg Sodium

191. Garganelli with Zucchini Pesto and Shrimp

Preparation Time: 10 minutes

Cook time: 30 minutes

Servings: 4

Ingredients

- 14 oz egg-based Garganelli
- For the zucchini pesto:
- 7oz Zucchini
- 1 cup Pine nuts
- 8 tablespoons (0.35oz) Basil
- 1 teaspoon of table Salt
- 9 tablespoons extra virgin olive oil
- 2 tablespoons Parmesan cheese to be grated
- 1oz of Pecorino to be grated
- For the sautéed shrimp:
- 8.8oz shrimp
- 1 clove garlic
- 7 teaspoons extra virgin olive oil
- Pinch of Salt

Directions

1. Start by preparing the pesto:
2. After washing the zucchini, grate them, place them in a colander (to allow them to lose some excess liquid), and lightly salt them. Put the pine nuts, zucchini and basil leaves in the blender. Add the grated Parmesan, the pecorino and the extra virgin olive oil.
3. Blend everything until the mixture is creamy, stir in a pinch of salt and set aside.
4. Switch to the shrimp:
5. First of all, pull out the intestine by cutting the shrimp's back with a knife along its entire length and, with the tip of the knife, remove the black thread inside.
6. Cook the clove of garlic in a non-stick pan with extra virgin olive oil. When its browned, remove the garlic and add the shrimps. Sauté them for about 5 minutes over medium heat, until you see a crispy crust form on the outside.
7. Then, boil a pot of salted water and cook the Garganelli. Set a couple of ladles of cooking water aside, and drain the pasta al dente.
8. Put the Garganelli in the pan where you cooked the shrimp. Cook together for a minute, add a ladle of cooking water and finally, add the zucchini pesto.
9. Mix everything well to combine the pasta with the sauce.

Nutrition (for 100g):

776 Calories

46g Fat

68g Carbohydrates

22.5g Protein

835mg Sodium

192.   Salmon Risotto

Preparation Time: 10 minutes

Cooking Time: 30 minutes

Serving: 4

Ingredients

- 1 ¾ cup (12.3 oz) of Rice
- 8.8oz Salmon steaks
- 1 Leek
- Extra virgin olive oil to taste
- 1 clove of garlic
- ½ glass white wine
- 3 ½ tablespoons grated Grana Padano
- salt to taste
- Black pepper to taste
- 17 fl. oz (500ml) Fish broth
- 1 cup butter

Directions

1. Start by cleaning the salmon and cutting it into small pieces. Cook 1 tablespoon of oil in a pan with a whole garlic clove and brown the salmon for 2/3 minutes, add salt and set the salmon aside, removing the garlic.
2. Now, start preparing the risotto:
3. Cut the leek into very small pieces and let it simmer in a pan over a low heat with two tablespoons of oil. Stir in the rice and cook it for a few seconds over medium-high heat, stirring with a wooden spoon.
4. Stir in the white wine and continue cooking, stirring occasionally, trying not to let the rice stick to the pan, and add the stock (vegetable or fish) gradually.
5. Halfway through cooking, add the salmon, butter, and a pinch of salt if necessary. When the rice is well cooked, remove from heat. Combine with a couple of tablespoons of grated Grana Padano and serve.

Nutrition (for 100g):

521 Calories

13g Fat

82g Carbohydrates

19g Protein

839mg Sodium

193.   Pasta with Cherry Tomatoes and Anchovies

Preparation Time: 15 minutes

Cooking Time: 35 minutes

Serving: 4

Ingredients

- 10.5oz Spaghetti
- 1.3-pound Cherry tomatoes
- 9oz Anchovies (pre-cleaned)
- 2 tablespoons Capers
- 1 clove of garlic
- 1 Small red onion
- Parsley to taste
- Extra virgin olive oil to taste
- Table salt to taste
- Black pepper to taste
- Black olives to taste

Directions

1. Cut the garlic clove, obtaining thin slices.
2. Cut the cherry tomatoes in 2. Peel the onion and slice it thinly.
3. Put a little oil with the sliced garlic and onions in a saucepan. Heat everything over medium heat for 5 minutes; stir occasionally.
4. Once everything has been well flavored, add the cherry tomatoes and a pinch of salt and pepper. Cook for 15 minutes. In the meantime, situate a pot with water on the stove and as soon as it boils, add the salt and the pasta.
5. Once the sauce is almost ready, mix in the anchovies and cook for a couple of minutes. Stir gently.
6. Turn off the heat, chop the parsley and place it in the pan.

7. When its cooked, strain the pasta and stir in directly to the sauce. Turn the heat back on again for a few seconds.

Nutrition (for 100g):

446 Calories

10g Fat

66.1g Carbohydrates

22.8g Protein

934mg Sodium

194. Broccoli and Sausage Orecchiette

Preparation Time: 10 minutes

Cooking Time: 32 minutes

Serving: 4

Ingredients

- 11.5oz Orecchiette
- Broccoli
- 10.5oz Sausage
- fl. oz(40ml) White wine
- 1 clove of garlic
- 2 sprigs of thyme
- 7 teaspoons extra virgin olive oil
- Black pepper to taste
- Table salt to taste

Directions

2. Boil the pot with full of water and salt. Remove the broccoli florets from the stalk and cut them in half or in 4 parts if they are too big; then, put them into the boiling water and covering the pot, cook for 6-7 minutes.
3. Meanwhile, finely chop thyme and set aside. Pull the gut from the sausage and with the help of a fork crush it gently.
4. Fry the garlic clove with a little olive oil and add the sausage. After a few seconds, add the thyme and a little white wine.
5. Without tossing out the cooking water, remove the cooked broccoli with the help of a slotted spoon and add them to the meat a little at a time. Cook everything for

3-4 minutes. Remove the garlic and add a pinch of black pepper.
6. Allow the water where you cooked the broccoli to reach a boil, then toss in the pasta and let it cook. Once the pasta is cooked, strain it with a slotted spoon, transferring it directly to the broccoli and sausage sauce. Then, mix well, adding black pepper and sautéing everything in the pan for a couple of minutes.

Nutrition (for 100g):

683 Calories

36g Fat

69.6g Carbohydrates

20g Protein

733mg Sodium

195. Radicchio and Smoked Bacon Risotto

Preparation Time: 10 minutes

Cooking Time: 30 minutes

Serving: 3

Ingredients

- 1 ½ cup of Rice
- 14oz Radicchio
- 5.3oz Smoked bacon
- 34 fl. oz (1l) Vegetable broth
- fl. oz(100ml) Red wine
- 7 teaspoons extra virgin olive oil
- 1.7oz Shallots
- Table salt to taste
- Black pepper to taste
- 3 sprigs of thyme

Directions

1. Let's begin with the preparation of the vegetable broth.
2. Start with the radicchio: cut it in half and remove the central part (the white part). Cut it into strips, rinse well and set it aside. Cut the smoked bacon into tiny strips as well.

3. Finely chop the shallot and situate it in a pan with a little oil. Let it simmer over medium heat, adding a ladle of broth, then, add the bacon and let it brown.
4. After about 2 minutes, add the rice and toast it, stirring often. At this point, pour the red wine over high heat.
5. Once all the alcohol has evaporated, continue cooking adding a ladle of broth at a time. Let the previous one dry before adding another, until fully cooked. Add salt and black pepper (it's up to how much you decide to add).
6. At the end of cooking, add the strips of radicchio. Mix them well until they are blended with the rice, but without cooking them. Add the chopped thyme.

Nutrition (for 100g):

482 Calories

17.5g Fat

68.1g Carbohydrates

13g Protein

725 mg Sodium

196.   Pasta ala Genovese

Preparation Time: 10 minutes

Cooking Time: 25 minutes

Serving: 3

Ingredients

- 11.5oz of Ziti
- 1 pound of Beef
  - pounds golden onions
- 2oz Celery
- 2oz Carrots
- 1 tuft of parsley
  - fl. oz(100ml) White wine
- Extra virgin olive oil to taste
- Table salt to taste
- Black pepper to taste
- Parmesan to taste

Directions

1. To prepare the pasta start by:

2. Peeling and finely chopping the onions and carrots. Then, wash and finely chop the celery (do not throw away the leaves, which must also be chopped and set aside). Next, switch to the meat, clean it of any excess fat and cut it into 5/6 large pieces. Finally, tie the celery leaves and parsley sprig with kitchen twine to create a fragrant bunch.
3. Fill plenty of oil in a large pan. Add the onions, celery, and carrots (which you had previously set aside) and let them cook for a couple of minutes.
4. Then, add the pieces of meat, a pinch of salt and the fragrant bunch. Stir and cook for a few minutes. Next, lower the heat and cover with a lid.
5. Cook for at least 3 hours (do not add water or broth because the onions will release all the liquid needed to prevent the bottom of the pan from drying). Occasionally, check on everything and stir.
6. After 3 hours of cooking, remove the bunch of herbs, increase the heat slightly, add a part of the wine and stir.
7. Cook the meat without a lid for about an hour, stirring often and adding the wine when the bottom of the pan dries.
8. At this point, take a piece of meat, cut it into slices on a cutting board and set aside. Chop the ziti and cook them in boiling salted water.
9. Once cooked, drain it and place it back in the pot. Dash a few tablespoons of cooking water and stir. Place on a plate and add a little sauce and crumbled meat (the one set aside in step 7). Add pepper and grated Parmesan to taste.

Nutrition (for 100g):

450 Calories

8g Fat

80g Carbohydrates

14.5g Protein

816mg Sodium

197. Cauliflower Pasta from Naples

Preparation Time: 15 minutes

Cooking Time: 35 minutes

Servings: 3

Ingredients

- o   oz Pasta
- 1 cauliflower
  - o   fl. oz (100 ml) of tomato puree
- 1 clove of garlic
- 1 chili pepper
- 3 tablespoons extra virgin olive oil (or teaspoons)
- Salt to taste
- Pepper to taste

Directions

1. Clean the cauliflower well: remove the outer leaves and the stalk. Cut it into small florets.
2. Peel the garlic clove, chop it and brown it in a saucepan with the oil and the chili pepper.
3. Add the tomato puree and cauliflower florets and let them brown for a few minutes over medium heat, then cover with a few ladles of water and cook for 15-20 minutes or at least until the cauliflower begins to become creamy.
4. If you see that the bottom of the pan is too dry, add as much water as needed so that the mixture remains liquid.
5. At this point, cover the cauliflower with hot water and, once it comes to a boil, add in the pasta.
6. Season with salt and pepper.

Nutrition (for 100g):

458 Calories

18g Fat

65g Carbohydrates

9g Protein

746mg Sodium

198. Pasta e Fagioli with Orange and Fennel

Preparation Time: 10 minutes

Cooking Time: 30 minutes

Servings: 5

Ingredients

- Extra-virgin olive oil – 1 tbsp. plus extra for serving
- Pancetta – 2 ounces, chopped fine
- Onion – 1, chopped fine
- Fennel – 1 bulb, stalks discarded, bulb halved, cored, and chopped fine
- Celery – 1 rib, minced
- Garlic – 2 cloves, minced
- Anchovy fillets – 3, rinsed and minced
- Minced fresh oregano – 1 tbsp.
- Grated orange zest – 2 tsp.
- Fennel seeds – ½ tsp.
- Red pepper flakes – ¼ tsp.
- Diced tomatoes – 1 (28-ounce) can
- Parmesan cheese – 1 rind, plus more for serving
- Cannellini beans – 1 (7-ounce) cans, rinsed
- Chicken broth – 2 ½ cups
- Water – 2 ½ cups
- Salt and pepper
- Orzo – 1 cup
- Minced fresh parsley – ¼ cup

Directions:

1. Heat oil in a Dutch oven over medium heat. Add pancetta. Stir-fry for 3 to 5 minutes or until beginning to brown. Stir in celery, fennel, and onion and stir-fry until softened (about 5 to 7 minutes).
2. Stir in pepper flakes, fennel seeds, orange zest, oregano, anchovies, and garlic. Cook for 1 minute. Stir in tomatoes and their juice. Stir in Parmesan rind and beans.
3. Simmer and cook for 10 minutes. Stir in water, broth, and 1 tsp. salt. Let it boil on high heat. Stir in pasta and cook until al dente.

4. Remove from heat and discard parmesan rind.
5. Stir in parsley and season with salt and pepper to taste. Pour some olive oil and topped with grated Parmesan. Serve.

Nutrition (for 100g):

502 Calories

8.8g Fat

72.2g Carbohydrates

34.9g Protein

693mg Sodium

199.   Spaghetti al Limone

Preparation Time: 10 minutes

Cooking Time: 15 minutes

Servings: 6

Ingredients

- Extra-virgin olive oil – ½ cup
- Grated lemon zest – 2 tsp.
- Lemon juice – 1/3 cup
- Garlic – 1 clove, minced to pate
- Salt and pepper
- Parmesan cheese – 2 ounces, grated
- Spaghetti – 1 pound
- Shredded fresh basil – 6 tbsp.

Directions:

1. In a bowl, whisk garlic, oil, lemon zest, juice, ½ tsp. salt and ¼ tsp. pepper. Stir in the Parmesan and mix until creamy.
2. Meanwhile, cook the pasta according to package directions. Drain and reserve ½ cup cooking water. Add the oil mixture and basil to the pasta and toss to combine. Season well and stir in the cooking water as needed. Serve.

Nutrition (for 100g):

398 Calories

20.7g Fat

42.5g Carbohydrates

11.9g Protein

844mg Sodium

200.   Spiced Vegetable Couscous

Preparation Time: 10 minutes

Cooking Time: 20 minutes

Servings: 6

Ingredients

- Cauliflower – 1 head, cut into 1 –inch florets
- Extra-virgin olive oil – 6 tbsp. plus extra for serving
- Salt and pepper
- Couscous – 1 ½ cups
- Zucchini – 1, cut into ½ inch pieces
- Red bell pepper – 1, stemmed, seeded, and cut into ½ inch pieces
- Garlic – 4 cloves, minced
- Ras el hanout – 2 tsp.
- Grated lemon zest -1 tsp. plus lemon wedges for serving
- Chicken broth – 1 ¾ cups
- Minced fresh marjoram – 1 tbsp.

Directions:

1. In a skillet, heat 2 tbsp. oil over medium heat. Add cauliflowers, ¾ tsp. salt, and ½ tsp. pepper. Mix. Cook until the florets turn brown and the edges are just translucent.
2. Remove the lid and cook, stirring for 10 minutes, or until the florets turn golden brown. Transfer to a bowl and clean the skillet. Heat 2 tbsp. oil in the skillet.
3. Add the couscous. Cook and continue stirring for 3 to 5 minutes, or until grains are just beginning to brown. Transfer to a bowl and clean the skillet. Heat the remaining 3 tbsp. oil in the skillet and add bell pepper, zucchini, and ½ tsp. salt. Cook for 8 minutes.
4. Stir in lemon zest, ras el hanout, and garlic. Cook until fragrant (about 30 seconds). Place in the broth and simmer. Stir in the couscous. Pull out from the heat, and set aside until tender.

5. Add marjoram and cauliflower; then gently fluff with a fork to incorporate. Drizzle with extra oil and season well. Serve with lemon wedges.

Nutrition (for 100g):

787 Calories

18.3g Fat

129.6g Carbohydrates

24.5g Protein

699mg Sodium

201.   Spiced Baked Rice with Fennel

Preparation Time: 10 minutes

Cooking Time: 45 minutes

Servings: 8

Ingredients

- Sweet potatoes – 1 ½ pounds, peeled and cut into 1-inch pieces
- Extra-virgin olive oil – ¼ cup
- Salt and pepper
- Fennel – 1 bulb, chopped fine
- Small onion – 1, chopped fine
- Long-grain white rice – 1 ½ cups, rinsed
- Garlic – 4 cloves, minced
- Ras el hanout – 2 tsp.
- Chicken broth – 2 ¾ cups
- Large pitted brine-cured green olives – ¾ cup, halved
- Minced fresh cilantro – 2 tbsp.
- Lime wedges

Directions:

1. Situate the oven rack to the middle and preheat oven to 400F. Toss the potatoes with ½ tsp. salt and 2 tbsp. oil.
2. Lay the potatoes in a single layer in a rimmed baking sheet and roast for 25 to 30 minutes, or until tender. Stir the potatoes halfway through roasting.
3. Pull out the potatoes and lower the oven temperature to 350F. In a Dutch oven,

heat the remaining 2 tbsp. oil over medium heat.
4. Add onion and fennel; next, cook for 5 to 7 minutes, or until softened. Stir in ras el hanout, garlic, and rice. Stir-fry for 3 minutes.
5. Stir in the olives and broth and let sit for 10 minutes. Add the potatoes to the rice and fluff gently with a fork to combine. Season with salt and pepper to taste. Garnish with cilantro and serve with lime wedges.

Nutrition (for 100g):

207 Calories

8.9g Fat

29.4g Carbohydrates

3.9g Protein

711mg Sodium

202.   Moroccan-Style Couscous with Chickpeas

Preparation Time: 5 minutes

Cooking Time: 18 minutes

Servings: 6

Ingredients

- Extra-virgin olive oil – ¼ cup, extra for serving
- Couscous – 1 ½ cups
- Peeled and chopped fine carrots – 2
- Chopped fine onion – 1
- Salt and pepper
- Garlic – 3 cloves, minced
- Ground coriander – 1 tsp.
- Ground ginger - tsp.
- Ground anise seed – ¼ tsp.
- Chicken broth – 1 ¾ cups
- Chickpeas - 1 (15-ounce) can, rinsed
- Frozen peas – 1 ½ cups
- Chopped fresh parsley or cilantro – ½ cup
- Lemon wedges

Directions:

1. Heat 2 tbsp. oil in a skillet over medium heat. Mix in the couscous and cook for 3 to 5 minutes, or until just beginning to brown. Transfer to a bowl and clean the skillet.
2. Heat remaining 2 tbsp. oil in the skillet and add the onion, carrots, and 1 tsp. salt. Cook for 5 to 7 minutes. Stir in anise, ginger, coriander, and garlic. Cook until fragrant (about 30 seconds).
3. Combine the chickpeas and broth and bring to simmer. Stir in the couscous and peas. Cover and remove from the heat. Set aside until the couscous is tender.
4. Add the parsley to the couscous and lint with a fork to combine. Dash with extra oil and season well. Serve with lemon wedges.

Nutrition (for 100g):

649 Calories

14.2g Fat

102.8g Carbohydrates

30.1g Protein

812mg Sodium

203. Vegetarian Paella with Green Beans and Chickpeas

Preparation Time: 10 minutes

Cooking Time: 35 minutes

Servings: 4

Ingredients

- Pinch of saffron
- Vegetable broth – 3 cups
- Olive oil – 1 tbsp.
- Yellow onion – 1 large, diced
- Garlic – 4 cloves, sliced
- Red bell pepper – 1, diced
- Crushed tomatoes – ¾ cup, fresh or canned
- Tomato paste – 2 tbsp.
- Hot paprika – 1 ½ tsp.

- Salt – 1 tsp.
- Freshly ground black pepper – ½ tsp.
- Green beans – 1 ½ cups, trimmed and halved
- Chickpeas – 1 (15-ounce) can, drained and rinsed
- Short-grain white rice – 1 cup
- Lemon – 1, cut into wedges

Directions:

1. Mix the saffron threads with 3 tbsp. warm water in a small bowl. In a saucepan, simmer the water over medium heat. Reduce the heat and allow to simmer.
2. Cook the oil in a skillet over medium heat. Mix in the onion and stir-fry for 5 minutes. Add the bell pepper and garlic and stir-fry for 7 minutes or until pepper is softened. Stir in the saffron-water mixture, salt, pepper, paprika, tomato paste, and tomatoes.
3. Add the rice, chickpeas, and green beans. Stir in the warm broth and bring to a boil. Lower the heat and simmer uncovered for 20 minutes.
4. Serve hot, garnished with lemon wedges.

Nutrition (for 100g):

709 Calories

12g Fat

121g Carbohydrates

33g Protein

633mg Sodium

204. Garlic Prawns with Tomatoes and Basil

Preparation Time: 10 minutes

Cooking Time: 10 minutes

Servings: 4

Ingredients

- Olive oil – 2 tbsp.
- Prawns – 1 ¼ pounds, peeled and deveined
- Garlic – 3 cloves, minced

- Crushed red pepper flakes – 1/8 tsp.
- Dry white wine – ¾ cup
- Grape tomatoes – 1 ½ cups
- Finely chopped fresh basil – ¼ cup, plus more for garnish
- Salt – ¾ tsp.
- Ground black pepper – ½ tsp.

Directions:

1. In a skillet, heat up the oil over medium-high heat. Add the prawns and cook for 1 minute, or until just cooked through. Transfer to a plate.
2. Place the red pepper flakes, and garlic to the oil in the pan and cook, stirring, for 30 seconds. Stir in the wine and cook until it's reduced by about half.
3. Add the tomatoes and stir-fry until tomatoes begin to break down (about 3 to 4 minutes). Stir in the reserved shrimp, salt, pepper, and basil. Cook for 1 to 2 minutes more.
4. Serve garnished with the remaining basil.

Nutrition (for 100g):

282 Calories

10g Fat

7g Carbohydrates

33g Protein

593mg Sodium

205.   Shrimp Paella

Preparation Time: 10 minutes

Cooking Time: 25 minutes

Servings: 4

Ingredients

- Olive oil – 2 tbsp.
- Medium onion – 1, diced
- Red bell pepper – 1, diced
- Garlic – 3 cloves, minced
- Pinch of saffron
- Hot paprika – ¼ tsp.
- Salt – 1 tsp.

- Freshly ground black pepper – ½ tsp.
- Chicken broth – 3 cups, divided
- Short-grain white rice - 1 cup
- Peeled and deveined large shrimp – 1 pound
- Frozen peas – 1 cup, thawed

Directions:

1. Heat olive oil in a skillet. Stir in the onion and bell pepper and stir-fry for 6 minutes, or until softened. Add the salt, pepper, paprika, saffron, and garlic and mix. Stir in 2 ½ cups of broth and rice.
2. Allow the mixture to boil, then simmer until the rice is cooked, about 12 minutes. Lay the shrimp and peas over the rice and add the remaining ½ cup broth.
3. Place the lid back on the skillet and cook until all shrimp are just cooked through (about 5 minutes). Serve.

Nutrition (for 100g):

409 Calories

10g Fat

51g Carbohydrates

25g Protein

693mg Sodium

206.   Lentil Salad with Olives, Mint, and Feta

Preparation Time: 1 hour

Cooking Time: 1 hour

Servings: 6

Ingredients

- Salt and pepper
- French lentils – 1 cup, picked over and rinsed
- Garlic – 5 cloves, lightly crushed and peeled
- Bay leaf – 1
- Extra-virgin olive oil – 5 tbsp.
- White wine vinegar – 3 tbsp.
- Pitted Kalamata olives – ½ cup, chopped

- Chopped fresh mint – ½ cup
- Shallot – 1 large, minced
- Feta cheese – 1 ounce, crumbled

Directions:

1. Add 4 cups warm water and 1 tsp. salt in a bowl. Add the lentils and soak at room temperature for 1 hour. Drain well.
2. Place the oven rack to the middle and heat the oven to 325F. Combine the lentils, 4 cups water, garlic, bay leaf, and ½ tsp. salt in a saucepan. Cover and situate the saucepan to the oven, and cook for 40 to 60 minutes, or until the lentils are tender.
3. Drain the lentils well, discarding garlic and bay leaf. In a large bowl, scourge oil and vinegar together. Add the shallot, mint, olives, and lentils and toss to combine.
4. Season with salt and pepper to taste. Place nicely in the serving dish and garnish with feta. Serve.

Nutrition (for 100g):

249 Calories

14.3g Fat

22.1g Carbohydrates

9.5g Protein

885mg Sodium

207.   Chickpeas with Garlic and Parsley

Preparation Time: 5 minutes

Cooking Time: 20 minutes

Servings: 6

Ingredients

- Extra-virgin olive oil – ¼ cup
- Garlic – 4 cloves, sliced thin
- Red pepper flakes – 1/8 tsp.
- Onion – 1, chopped
- Salt and pepper
- Chickpeas – 2 (15-ounce) cans, rinsed
- Chicken broth – 1 cup

- Minced fresh parsley – 2 tbsp.
- Lemon juice – 2 tsp.

Directions:

1. In a skillet, add 3 tbsp. oil and cook garlic, and pepper flakes for 3 minutes. Stir in onion and ¼ tsp. salt and cook for 5 to 7 minutes.
2. Mix in the chickpeas and broth and bring to a simmer. Lower heat and simmer on low heat for 7 minutes, covered.
3. Uncover and set the heat to high and cook for 3 minutes, or until all liquid has evaporated. Set aside and mix in the lemon juice and parsley.
4. Season with salt and pepper to taste. Drizzle with 1 tbsp. oil and serve.

Nutrition (for 100g):

611 Calories

17.6g Fat

89.5g Carbohydrates

28.7g Protein

789mg Sodium

208.   Stewed Chickpeas with Eggplant and Tomatoes

Preparation Time: 10 minutes

Cooking Time: 1 hour

Servings: 6

Ingredients

- Extra-virgin olive oil – ¼ cup
- Onions – 2, chopped
- Green bell pepper – 1, chopped fine
- Salt and pepper
- Garlic – 3 cloves, minced
- Minced fresh oregano – 1 tbsp.
- Bay leaves – 2
- Eggplant – 1 pound, cut into 1-inch pieces
- Whole peeled tomatoes – 1, can, drained with juice reserved, chopped

- Chickpeas – 2(15-ounce) cans, drained with 1 cup liquid reserved

Directions:

1. Situate the oven rack on the lower-middle part and heat the oven to 400F. Heat oil in the Dutch oven. Add bell pepper, onions, ½ tsp. salt, and ¼ tsp. pepper. Stir-fry for 5 minutes.
2. Stir in 1 tsp. oregano, garlic, and bay leaves and cook for 30 seconds. Stir in tomatoes, eggplant, reserved juice, chickpeas, and reserved liquid and bring to a boil. Transfer the pot to oven and cook, uncovered, for 45 to 60 minutes. Stirring twice.
3. Discard the bay leaves. Stir in the remaining 2 tsp. oregano and season with salt and pepper. Serve.

Nutrition (for 100g):

642 Calories

17.3g Fat

93.8g Carbohydrates

29.3g Protein

983mg Sodium

209. Greek Lemon Rice

Preparation Time: 20 minutes

Cooking Time: 45 minutes

Servings: 6

Ingredients

- Long grain rice – 2 cups, uncooked (soaked in cold water for 20 minutes, then drained)
- Extra virgin olive oil – 3 tbsp.
- Yellow onion – 1 medium, chopped
- Garlic - 1 clove, minced
- Orzo pasta – ½ cup
- Juice of 2 lemons, plus zest of 1 lemon
- Low sodium broth – 2 cups
- Pinch salt
- Chopped parsley – 1 large handful

- Dill weed – 1 tsp.

Directions:

1. In a saucepan, heat 3 tbsp. extra virgin olive oil. Add the onions and stir-fry for 3 to 4 minutes. Add the orzo pasta and garlic and toss to mix.
2. Then toss in the rice to coat. Add the broth and lemon juice. Bring to a boil and lower the heat. Cover and cook for about 20 minutes.
3. Remove from the heat. Cover and set aside for 10 minutes. Uncover and stir in the lemon zest, dill weed, and parsley. Serve.

Nutrition (for 100g):

145 Calories

6.9g Fat

18.3g Carbohydrates

3.3g Protein

893mg Sodium

210. Garlic-Herb Rice

Preparation Time: 10 minutes

Cooking Time: 30 minutes

Servings: 4

Ingredients

- Extra-virgin olive oil – ½ cup, divided
- Large garlic cloves – 5, minced
- Brown jasmine rice – 2 cups
- Water – 4 cups
- Sea salt – 1 tsp.
- Black pepper – 1 tsp.
- Chopped fresh chives – 3 tbsp.
- Chopped fresh parsley – 2 tbsp.
- Chopped fresh basil – 1 tbsp.

Directions:

1. In a saucepan, add ¼-cup olive oil, garlic, and rice. Stir and heat over medium heat. Stir in the water, sea salt, and black pepper. Next, mix again.

2. Bring to a boil and lower the heat. Simmer, uncovered, stirring occasionally.
3. When the water is almost absorbed, mix the remaining ¼-cup olive oil, along with the basil, parsley, and chives.
4. Stir until the herbs are incorporated and all the water is absorbed.

Nutrition (for 100g):

304 Calories

25.8g Fat

19.3g Carb

2g Protein

874mg Sodium

211. Mediterranean Rice Salad

Preparation Time: 10 minutes

Cooking Time: 25 minutes

Servings: 4

Ingredients

- Extra virgin olive oil – ½ cup, divided
- Long-grain brown rice – 1 cup
- Water – 2 cups
- Fresh lemon juice – ¼ cup
- Garlic clove – 1, minced
- Minced fresh rosemary – 1 tsp.
- Minced fresh mint – 1 tsp.
- Belgian endives – 3, chopped
- Red bell pepper – 1 medium, chopped
- Hothouse cucumber – 1, chopped
- Chopped whole green onion – ½ cup
- Chopped Kalamata olives – ½ cup
- Red pepper flakes – ¼ tsp.
- Crumbled feta cheese – ¾ cup
- Sea salt and black pepper

Directions:

1. Heat ¼-cup olive oil, rice, and a pinch of salt in a saucepan over low heat. Stir to coat the rice. Add the water and let simmer until the water is absorbed. Stirring occasionally. Pour the rice into a large bowl and cool.

2. In another bowl, mix together the remaining ¼ cup olive oil, red pepper flakes, olives, green onion, cucumber, bell pepper, endives, mint, rosemary, garlic, and lemon juice.
3. Place the rice to the mixture and toss to combine. Gently mix in the feta cheese.
4. Taste and adjust the seasoning. Serve.

Nutrition (for 100g):

415 Calories

34g Fat

28.3g Carbohydrates

7g Protein

4755mg Sodium

212. Fresh Bean and Tuna Salad

Preparation Time: 5 minutes

Cooking Time: 20 minutes

Servings: 6

Ingredients

- Shelled (shucked) fresh beans – 2 cups
- Bay leaves – 2
- Extra-virgin olive oil – 3 tbsp.
- Red wine vinegar – 1 tbsp.
- Salt and black pepper
- Best-quality tuna - 1 (6-ounce) can, packed in olive oil
- Salted capers – 1 tbsp. soaked and dried
- Finely minced flat-leaf parsley – 2 tbsp.
- Red onion – 1, sliced

Directions:

1. Boil lightly salted water in a pot. Add the beans and bay leaves; next, cook for 15 to 20 minutes, or until the beans are tender but still firm. Drain, discard aromatics, and transfer to a bowl.
2. Immediately dress the beans with vinegar and oil. Add the salt and black pepper. Mix well and adjust seasoning. Drain the tuna and flake the tuna flesh into the bean salad. Add the parsley and capers. Toss to

mix and scatter the red onion slices over the top. Serve.

Nutrition (for 100g):

85 Calories

7.1g Fat

4.7g Carbohydrates

1.8g Protein

863mg Sodium

213. Delicious Chicken Pasta

Preparation Time: 10 minutes

Cooking Time: 17 minutes

Serving: 4

Ingredients:

- 3 chicken breasts, skinless, boneless, cut into pieces
- 9 oz whole-grain pasta
- 1/2 cup olives, sliced
- 1/2 cup sun-dried tomatoes
- 1 tbsp roasted red peppers, chopped
- 14 oz can tomato, diced
- 2 cups marinara sauce
- 1 cup chicken broth
- Pepper
- Salt

Directions:

1. Stir in all ingredients except whole-grain pasta into the instant pot.
2. Seal the lid and cook on high for 12 minutes.
3. Once done, allow to release pressure naturally. Remove lid.
4. Add pasta and stir well. Seal pot again and select manual and set timer for 5 minutes.
5. When finished, release the pressure for 5 minutes then release remaining using quick release. Remove lid. Stir well and serve.

Nutrition (for 100g):

615 Calories

15.4g Fat

71g Carbohydrates

48g Protein

631mg Sodium

214. Flavors Taco Rice Bowl

Preparation Time: 10 minutes

Cooking Time: 14 minutes

Serving: 8

Ingredients:

- 1 lb. ground beef
- 8 oz cheddar cheese, shredded
- 14 oz can red beans
- 2 oz taco seasoning
- 16 oz salsa
- 2 cups of water
- 2 cups brown rice
- Pepper
- Salt

Directions:

1. Set instant pot on sauté mode.
2. Add meat to the pot and sauté until brown.
3. Add water, beans, rice, taco seasoning, pepper, and salt and stir well.
4. Top with salsa. Close the lid and cook on high for 14 minutes.
5. Once done, release pressure using quick release. Remove lid.
6. Mix in the cheddar cheese and stir until cheese is melted.
7. Serve and enjoy.

Nutrition (for 100g):

464 Calories

15.3g Fat

48.9g Carbohydrates

32.2g Protein

612mg Sodium

215. Flavorful Mac & Cheese

Preparation Time: 10 minutes

Cooking Time: 10 minutes

Serving: 6

Ingredients:

- 16 oz whole-grain elbow pasta
- 4 cups of water
- 1 cup can tomato, diced
- 1 tsp garlic, chopped
- 2 tbsp olive oil
- 1/4 cup green onions, chopped
- 1/2 cup parmesan cheese, grated
- 1/2 cup mozzarella cheese, grated
- 1 cup cheddar cheese, grated
- 1/4 cup passata
- 1 cup unsweetened almond milk
- 1 cup marinated artichoke, diced
- 1/2 cup sun-dried tomatoes, sliced
- 1/2 cup olives, sliced
- 1 tsp salt

Directions:

1. Add pasta, water, tomatoes, garlic, oil, and salt into the instant pot and stir well. Cover lid and cook on high.
2. Once done, release pressure for few minutes then releases remaining using quick discharge. Remove lid.
3. Set pot on sauté mode. Add green onion, parmesan cheese, mozzarella cheese, cheddar cheese, passata, almond milk, artichoke, sun-dried tomatoes, and olive. Mix well.
4. Stir well and cook until cheese is melted.
1. Serve and enjoy.

Nutrition (for 100g):

519 Calories

17.1g Fat

66.5g Carbohydrates

25g Protein

588mg Sodium

216. Cucumber Olive Rice

Preparation Time: 10 minutes

Cooking Time: 10 minutes

Serving: 8

Ingredients:

- 2 cups rice, rinsed
- 1/2 cup olives, pitted
- 1 cup cucumber, chopped
- 1 tbsp red wine vinegar
- 1 tsp lemon zest, grated
- 1 tbsp fresh lemon juice
- 2 tbsp olive oil
- 2 cups vegetable broth
- 1/2 tsp dried oregano
- 1 red bell pepper, chopped
- 1/2 cup onion, chopped
- 1 tbsp olive oil
- Pepper
- Salt

Directions:

2. Add oil into the inner pot of instant pot and select the pot on sauté mode. Add onion and sauté for 3 minutes. Add bell pepper and oregano and sauté for 1 minute.
3. Add rice and broth and stir well. Seal the lid and cook on high for 6 minutes. Once done, allow pressure release for 10 minutes then release remaining using quick release. Remove lid.
4. Add remaining ingredients and stir everything well to mix. Serve immediately and enjoy it.

Nutrition (for 100g):

229 Calories

5.1g Fat

40.2g Carbohydrates

4.9g Protein

210mg Sodium

217. Flavors Herb Risotto

Preparation Time: 10 minutes

Cooking Time: 15 minutes

Serving: 4

Ingredients:

- 2 cups of rice
- 2 tbsp parmesan cheese, grated
  - oz heavy cream
- 1 tbsp fresh oregano, chopped
- 1 tbsp fresh basil, chopped
- 1/2 tbsp sage, chopped
- 1 onion, chopped
- 2 tbsp olive oil
- 1 tsp garlic, minced
- 4 cups vegetable stock
- Pepper
- Salt

Directions:

1. Add oil into the inner vessel of instant pot and click the pot on sauté mode. Add garlic and onion the inner pan of instant pot and press the pot on sauté mode. Add garlic and onion and sauté for 2-3 minutes.
2. Add remaining ingredients except for parmesan cheese and heavy cream and stir well. Seal lid and cook on high for 12 minutes.
3. Once done, discharge the pressure for 10 minutes then release remaining using quick release. Remove lid. Stir in cream and cheese and serve.

Nutrition (for 100g):

514 Calories

17.6g Fat

79.4g Carbohydrates

8.8g Protein

488mg Sodium

218. Delicious Pasta Primavera

Preparation Time: 10 minutes

Cooking Time: 4 minutes

Serving: 4

Ingredients:

- 8 oz whole wheat penne pasta
- 1 tbsp fresh lemon juice
- 2 tbsp fresh parsley, chopped
- 1/4 cup almonds slivered
- 1/4 cup parmesan cheese, grated
- 14 oz can tomato, diced
- 1/2 cup prunes
- 1/2 cup zucchini, chopped
- 1/2 cup asparagus
- 1/2 cup carrots, chopped
- 1/2 cup broccoli, chopped
- 1 3/4 cups vegetable stock
- Pepper
- Salt

Directions:

1. Add stock, pars, tomatoes, prunes, zucchini, asparagus, carrots, and broccoli into the instant pot and stir well. Close and cook on high for 4 minutes. Once done, release pressure using quick release. Take out lid. Stir remaining ingredients well and serve.

Nutrition (for 100g):

303 Calories

2.6g Fat

63.5g Carbohydrates

12.8g Protein

918mg Sodium

219. Roasted Pepper Pasta

Preparation Time: 10 minutes

Cooking Time: 13 minutes

Serving: 6

Ingredients:

- 1 lb. whole wheat penne pasta
- 1 tbsp Italian seasoning
- 4 cups vegetable broth
- 1 tbsp garlic, minced
- 1/2 onion, chopped
- 14 oz jar roasted red peppers
- 1 cup feta cheese, crumbled
- 1 tbsp olive oil
- Pepper
- Salt

Directions:

2. Add roasted pepper into the blender and blend until smooth. Add oil into the inner pot of instant pot and set the jug on sauté mode. Add garlic and onion the inner cup of instant pot and set the pot on sauté. Add garlic and onion and sauté for 2-3 minutes.
3. Add blended roasted pepper and sauté for 2 minutes.
4. Add remaining ingredients except feta cheese and stir well. Seal it tight and cook on high for 8 minutes. When done, release pressure naturally for 5 minutes then releases the remaining using quick release. Remove lid. Top with feta cheese and serve.

Nutrition (for 100g):

459 Calories

10.6g Fat

68.1g Carbohydrates

21.3g Protein

724 mg Sodium

220. Cheese Basil Tomato Rice

Preparation Time: 10 minutes

Cooking Time: 26 minutes

Serving: 8

Ingredients:

- 1 1/2 cups brown rice

- 1 cup parmesan cheese, grated
- 1/4 cup fresh basil, chopped
- 2 cups grape tomatoes, halved
- 8 oz can tomato sauce
- 1 3/4 cup vegetable broth
- 1 tbsp garlic, minced
- 1/2 cup onion, diced
- 1 tbsp olive oil
- Pepper
- Salt

Directions:

1. Add oil into the inner basin of instant pot and select the pot on sauté. Put garlic and onion the inner vessel of instant pot and set it on sauté manner. Mix in garlic and onion and sauté for 4 minutes. Add rice, tomato sauce, broth, pepper, and salt and stir well.
2. Seal it and cook on high for 22 minutes.
3. Once done, let it release pressure for 10 minutes then release remaining using quick release. Remove cap. Stir in remaining ingredients and mix. Serve and enjoy.

Nutrition (for 100g):

208 Calories

5.6g Fat

32.1g Carbohydrates

8.3g Protein

863mg Sodium

221. Mac & Cheese

Preparation Time: 10 minutes

Cooking Time: 4 minutes

Serving: 8

Ingredients:

- 1 lb. whole grain pasta
- 1/2 cup parmesan cheese, grated
- 4 cups cheddar cheese, shredded
- 1 cup milk
- 1/4 tsp garlic powder

- 1/2 tsp ground mustard
- 2 tbsp olive oil
- 4 cups of water
- Pepper
- Salt

Directions:

1. Add pasta, garlic powder, mustard, oil, water, pepper, and salt into the instant pot. Seal tight and cook on high for 4 minutes. When done, release pressure using quick release. Open lid. Put remaining ingredients and stir well and serve.

Nutrition (for 100g):

509 Calories

25.7g Fat

43.8g Carbohydrates

27.3g Protein

766 mg Sodium

222. Tuna Pasta

Preparation Time: 10 minutes

Cooking Time: 8 minutes

Serving: 6

Ingredients:

- 10 oz can tuna, drained
- 15 oz whole wheat rotini pasta
- 4 oz mozzarella cheese, cubed
- 1/2 cup parmesan cheese, grated
- 1 tsp dried basil
- 14 oz can tomato
- 4 cups vegetable broth
- 1 tbsp garlic, minced
- 8 oz mushrooms, sliced
- 2 zucchinis, sliced
- 1 onion, chopped
- 2 tbsp olive oil
- Pepper
- Salt

Directions:

2. Pour oil into the inner pot of instant pot and press the pot on sauté. Add mushrooms, zucchini, and onion and sauté until onion is softened. Add garlic and sauté for a minute.
3. Add pasta, basil, tuna, tomatoes, and broth and stir well. Seal and cook on high for 4 minutes. When completed, release pressure for 5 minutes then releases the remaining using quick release. Remove lid. Add remaining ingredients and stir well and serve.

Nutrition (for 100g):

346 Calories

11.9g Fat

31.3g Carbohydrates

6.3g Protein

830mg Sodium

Poultry

223.   Chicken with Caper Sauce

Preparation Time: 20 minutes

Cooking Time: 18 minutes

Servings: 5

Ingredients:

- For Chicken:
- 2 eggs
- Salt and ground black pepper, as required
- 1 cup dry breadcrumbs
- 2 tablespoons olive oil
- 1½ pounds skinless, boneless chicken breast halves, pounded into ¾inch thickness and cut into pieces
- For Capers Sauce:
- 3 tablespoons capers
- ½ cup dry white wine
- 3 tablespoons fresh lemon juice
- Salt and ground black pepper, as required
- 2 tablespoons fresh parsley, chopped

Directions:

1. For chicken: in a shallow dish, add the eggs, salt and black pepper and beat until well combined. In another shallow dish, place breadcrumbs. Soak the chicken pieces in egg mixture then coat with the breadcrumbs evenly. Shake off the excess breadcrumbs.
2. Cook the oil over medium heat and cook the chicken pieces for about 5-7 minutes per side or until desired doneness. With a slotted spoon, situate the chicken pieces onto a paper towel lined plate. With a piece of the foil, cover the chicken pieces to keep them warm.
3. In the same skillet, incorporate all the sauce ingredients except parsley and cook for about 2-3 minutes, stirring continuously. Mix in the parsley and remove from heat. Serve the chicken pieces with the topping of capers sauce.

Nutrition (for 100g):

352 Calories

13.5g Fat

1.9g Carbohydrates

1.2g Protein

741mg Sodium

224.   Turkey Burgers with Mango Salsa

Preparation Time: 15 minutes

Cooking Time: 10 minutes

Servings: 6

Ingredients:

- 1½ pounds ground turkey breast
- 1 teaspoon sea salt, divided
- ¼ teaspoon freshly ground black pepper
- 2 tablespoons extra-virgin olive oil
- 2 mangos, peeled, pitted, and cubed
- ½ red onion, finely chopped
- Juice of 1 lime
- 1 garlic clove, minced
- ½ jalapeño pepper, seeded and finely minced
- 2 tablespoons chopped fresh cilantro leaves

Directions:

1. Form the turkey breast into 4 patties and season with ½ teaspoon of sea salt and the pepper. Cook the olive oil in a nonstick skillet until it shimmers. Add the turkey patties and cook for about 5 minutes per side until browned. While the patties cook, mix together the mango, red onion, lime juice, garlic, jalapeño, cilantro, and remaining ½ teaspoon of sea salt in a small bowl. Spoon the salsa over the turkey patties and serve.

Nutrition (for 100g):

384 Calories

3g Fat

27g Carbohydrates

34g Protein

692mg Sodium

225. One-Pan Tuscan Chicken

Preparation Time: 10 minutes

Cooking Time: 25 minutes

Servings: 6

Ingredients:

- ¼ cup extra-virgin olive oil, divided
- 1-pound boneless, skinless chicken breasts, cut into ¾-inch pieces
- 1 onion, chopped
- 1 red bell pepper, chopped
- 3 garlic cloves, minced
- ½ cup dry white wine
- 1 (14-ounce) can crushed tomatoes, undrained
- 1 (14-ounce) can chopped tomatoes, drained
- 1 (14-ounce) can white beans, drained
- 1 tablespoon dried Italian seasoning
- ½ teaspoon sea salt
- 1/8 teaspoon freshly ground black pepper
- 1/8 teaspoon red pepper flakes
- ¼ cup chopped fresh basil leaves

Directions:

1. Cook 2 tablespoons of olive oil until it shimmers. Mix in the chicken and cook until browned. Remove the chicken from the skillet and set aside on a platter, tented with aluminum foil to keep warm.
2. Situate the skillet back to the heat and heat up the remaining olive oil. Add the onion and red bell pepper. Cook and stir rarely, until the vegetables are soft. Put the garlic and cook for 30 seconds, stirring constantly.
3. Stir in the wine, and use the side of the spoon to scoop out any browned bits from the bottom of the pan. Cook for 1 minute, stirring.
4. Mix in the crushed and chopped tomatoes, white beans, Italian seasoning, sea salt, pepper, and red pepper flakes. Allow to simmer. Cook for 5 minutes, stirring occasionally.
5. Put the chicken back and any juices that have collected to the skillet. Cook until

the chicken is cook through. Take out from the heat and stir in the basil before serving.

Nutrition (for 100g):

271 Calories

8g Fat

29g Carbohydrates

14g Protein

596mg Sodium

226. Chicken Kapama

Preparation Time: 10 minutes

Cooking Time: 2 hours

Servings: 4

Ingredients:

- 1 (32-ounce) can chopped tomatoes, drained
- ¼ cup dry white wine
- 2 tablespoons tomato paste
- 3 tablespoons extra-virgin olive oil
- ¼ teaspoon red pepper flakes
- 1 teaspoon ground allspice
- ½ teaspoon dried oregano
- 2 whole cloves
- 1 cinnamon stick
- ½ teaspoon sea salt
- 1/8 teaspoon freshly ground black pepper
- 4 boneless, skinless chicken breast halves

Directions:

1. Mix the tomatoes, wine, tomato paste, olive oil, red pepper flakes, allspice, oregano, cloves, cinnamon stick, sea salt, and pepper in large pot. Bring to a simmer, stirring occasionally. Allow to simmer for 30 minutes, stirring occasionally. Remove and discard the whole cloves and cinnamon stick from the sauce and let the sauce cool.
2. Preheat the oven to 350°F. Situate the chicken in a 9-by-13-inch baking dish. Pour the sauce over the chicken and

cover the pan with aluminum foil. Continue baking until it reaches 165°F internal temperature.

Nutrition (for 100g):

220 Calories

3g Fat

11g Carbohydrates

8g Protein

923mg Sodium

227.   Spinach and Feta–Stuffed Chicken Breasts

Preparation Time: 10 minutes

Cooking Time: 45 minutes

Servings: 4

Ingredients:

- 2 tablespoons extra-virgin olive oil
- 1-pound fresh baby spinach
- 3 garlic cloves, minced
- Zest of 1 lemon
- ½ teaspoon sea salt
- 1/8 teaspoon freshly ground black pepper
- ½ cup crumbled feta cheese
- 4 boneless, skinless chicken breasts

Directions:

1. Preheat the oven to 350°F. Cook the olive oil over medium heat until it shimmers. Add the spinach. Continue cooking and stirring, until wilted.
2. Stir in the garlic, lemon zest, sea salt, and pepper. Cook for 30 seconds, stirring constantly. Cool slightly and mix in the cheese.
3. Spread the spinach and cheese mixture in an even layer over the chicken pieces and roll the breast around the filling. Hold closed with toothpicks or butcher's twine. Place the breasts in a 9-by-13-inch baking dish and bake for 30 to 40 minutes, or until the chicken have an internal temperature of 165°F. Take out from the

oven and set aside for 5 minutes before slicing and serving.

Nutrition (for 100g):

263 Calories

3g Fat

7g Carbohydrates

17g Protein

639mg Sodium

228.   Rosemary Baked Chicken Drumsticks

Preparation Time: 5 minutes

Cooking Time: 1 hour

Servings: 6

Ingredients:

- 2 tablespoons chopped fresh rosemary leaves
- 1 teaspoon garlic powder
- ½ teaspoon sea salt
- 1/8 teaspoon freshly ground black pepper
- Zest of 1 lemon
- 12 chicken drumsticks

Directions:

1. Preheat the oven to 350°F. Mix the rosemary, garlic powder, sea salt, pepper, and lemon zest.
2. Situate the drumsticks in a 9-by-13-inch baking dish and sprinkle with the rosemary mixture. Bake until the chicken reaches an internal temperature of 165°F.

Nutrition (for 100g):

163 Calories

1g Fat

2g Carbohydrates

26g Protein

633mg Sodium

229. Chicken with Onions, Potatoes, Figs, and Carrots

Preparation Time: 5 minutes

Cooking Time: 45 minutes

Servings: 4

Ingredients:

- 2 cups fingerling potatoes, halved
- 4 fresh figs, quartered
- 2 carrots, julienned
- 2 tablespoons extra-virgin olive oil
- 1 teaspoon sea salt, divided
- ¼ teaspoon freshly ground black pepper
- 4 chicken leg-thigh quarters
- 2 tablespoons chopped fresh parsley leaves

Directions:

1. Preheat the oven to 425°F. In a small bowl, toss the potatoes, figs, and carrots with the olive oil, ½ teaspoon of sea salt, and the pepper. Spread in a 9-by-13-inch baking dish.
2. Season the chicken with the rest of t sea salt. Place it on top of the vegetables. Bake until the vegetables are soft and the chicken reaches an internal temperature of 165°F. Sprinkle with the parsley and serve.

Nutrition (for 100g):

429 Calories

4g Fat

27g Carbohydrates

52g Protein

581mg Sodium

230. Moussaka

Preparation Time: 10 minutes

Cooking Time: 45 minutes

Servings: 8

Ingredients:

- 5 tablespoons extra-virgin olive oil, divided
- 1 eggplant, sliced (unpeeled)
- 1 onion, chopped
- 1 green bell pepper, seeded and chopped
- 1-pound ground turkey
- 3 garlic cloves, minced
- 2 tablespoons tomato paste
- 1 (14-ounce) can chopped tomatoes, drained
- 1 tablespoon Italian seasoning
- 2 teaspoons Worcestershire sauce
- 1 teaspoon dried oregano
- ½ teaspoon ground cinnamon
- 1 cup unsweetened nonfat plain Greek yogurt
- 1 egg, beaten
- ¼ teaspoon freshly ground black pepper
- ¼ teaspoon ground nutmeg
- ¼ cup grated Parmesan cheese
- 2 tablespoons chopped fresh parsley leaves

Directions:

1. Preheat the oven to 400°F. Cook 3 tablespoons of olive oil until it shimmers. Add the eggplant slices and brown for 3 to 4 minutes per side. Transfer to paper towels to drain.
2. Return the skillet back to the heat and pour the remaining 2 tablespoons of olive oil. Add the onion and green bell pepper. Continue cooking until the vegetables are soft. Remove from the pan and set aside.
3. Pull out the skillet to the heat and stir in the turkey. Cook for about 5 minutes, crumbling with a spoon, until browned. Stir in the garlic and cook for 30 seconds, stirring constantly.
4. Stir in the tomato paste, tomatoes, Italian seasoning, Worcestershire sauce, oregano, and cinnamon. Place the onion and bell pepper back to the pan. Cook for 5 minutes, stirring. Combine the yogurt, egg, pepper, nutmeg, and cheese.
5. Arrange half of the meat mixture in a 9-by-13-inch baking dish. Layer with half the eggplant. Add the remaining meat mixture and the remaining eggplant.

Spread with the yogurt mixture. Bake until golden brown. Garnish with the parsley and serve.

Nutrition (for 100g):

338 Calories

5g Fat

16g Carbohydrates

28g Protein

569mg Sodium

231.   Chicken in Tomato-Balsamic Pan Sauce

Preparation Time: 10 minutes

Cooking Time: 20 minutes

Servings: 4

Ingredients

- 2 (8 oz. or 226.7 g each) boneless chicken breasts, skinless
- ½ tsp. salt
- ½ tsp. ground pepper
- 3 tbsps. extra-virgin olive oil
- ½ c. halved cherry tomatoes
- 2 tbsps. sliced shallot
- ¼ c. balsamic vinegar
- 1 tbsp. minced garlic
- 1 tbsp. toasted fennel seeds, crushed
- 1 tbsp. butter

Directions;

1. Slice the chicken breasts into 4 pieces and beat them with a mallet till it reaches a thickness of a ¼ inch. Use ¼ teaspoons of pepper and salt to coat the chicken. Heat two tablespoons of oil in a skillet and keep the heat to a medium. Cook the chicken breasts on both sides for three minutes. Place it to a serving plate and cover it with foil to keep it warm.
2. Add one tablespoon oil, shallot, and tomatoes in a pan and cook till it softens. Add vinegar and boil the mix till the vinegar gets reduced by half. Put fennel

seeds, garlic, salt, and pepper and cook for about four minutes. Pull it out from the heat and stir it with butter.   Pour this sauce over chicken and serve.

Nutrition (for 100g):

294 Calories

17g Fat

10g Carbohydrates

 2g Protein

639mg Sodium

232.   Seasoned Buttered Chicken

Preparation Time: 10 minutes

Cooking Time: 20 minutes

Servings: 4

Ingredients

- ½ c. Heavy Whipping Cream
- 1 tbsp. Salt
- ½ c. Bone Broth
- 1 tbsp. Pepper
- 4 tbsps. Butter
- 4 Chicken Breast Halves

Directions:

1. Place cooking pan on your oven over medium heat and add in one tablespoon of butter. Once the butter is warm and melted, place the chicken in and cook for five minutes on either side. At the end of this time, the chicken should be cooked through and golden; if it is, go ahead and place it on a plate.
2. Next, you are going to add the bone broth into the warm pan. Add heavy whipping cream, salt, and pepper. Then, leave the pan alone until your sauce begins to simmer. Allow this process to happen for five minutes to let the sauce thicken up.
3. Finally, you are going to add the rest of your butter and the chicken back into the pan. Be sure to use a spoon to place the

sauce over your chicken and smother it completely. Serve

Nutrition (for 100g):

350 Calories

25g Fat

10g Carbohydrates

25g Protein

869mg Sodium

233. Double Cheesy Bacon Chicken

Preparation Time: 10 minutes

Cooking Time: 30 minutes

Servings: 4

Ingredients

- 4 oz. or 113 g. Cream Cheese
- 1 c. Cheddar Cheese
- 8 strips Bacon
- Sea salt
- Pepper
- 2 Garlic cloves, finely chopped
- Chicken Breast
- 1 tbsp. Bacon Grease or Butter

Directions:

1. Ready the oven to 400 F/204 C Slice the chicken breasts in half to make them thin
2. Season with salt, pepper, and garlic Grease a baking pan with butter and place chicken breasts into it. Add the cream cheese and cheddar cheese on top of the breasts
3. Add bacon slices as well Place the pan to the oven for 30 minutes Serve hot

Nutrition (for 100g):

610 Calories

32g Fat

3g Carbohydrates

38g Protein

759mg Sodium

234. Chili Oregano Baked Cheese

Preparation Time: 10 minutes

Cooking Time: 25 minutes

Servings: 4

Ingredients

- 8 oz. or 226.7g feta cheese
- 4 oz. or 113g mozzarella, crumbled
- 1 sliced chili pepper
- 1 tsp. dried oregano
- 2 tbsps. olive oil

Directions:

1. Place the feta cheese in a small deep-dish baking pan. Top with the mozzarella then season with pepper slices and oregano. cover your pan with lid. Bake in the preheated oven at 350 F/176 C for 20 minutes. Serve the cheese and enjoy it.

Nutrition (for 100g):

292 Calories

24.2g Fat

5.7g Carbohydrates

2g Protein

733mg Sodium

235. Crispy Italian Chicken

Preparation Time: 10 minutes

Cooking Time: 30 minutes

Servings: 4

Ingredients

- 4 chicken legs
- 1 tsp. dried basil
- 1 tsp. dried oregano
- Salt and pepper
- 3 tbsps. olive oil
- 1 tbsp. balsamic vinegar

Directions:

2. Season the chicken well with basil, and oregano. Using a skillet, add oil and heat. Add the chicken in the hot oil. Let each side cook for 5 minutes until golden then cover the skillet with a lid.
3. Adjust your heat to medium and cook for 10 minutes on one side then flip the chicken repeatedly, cooking for another 10 minutes until crispy. Serve the chicken and enjoy.

Nutrition (for 100g):

262 Calories

13.9g Fat

11g Carbohydrates

32.6g Protein

693mg Sodium

236.   Sea Bass in a Pocket

Preparation Time: 10 minutes

Cooking Time: 25 minutes

Servings: 4

Ingredients

- 4 sea bass fillets
- 4 sliced garlic cloves
- 1 sliced celery stalk
- 1 sliced zucchini
- 1 c. halved cherry tomatoes halved
- 1 shallot, sliced
- 1 tsp. dried oregano
- Salt and pepper

Directions:

1. Mix the garlic, celery, zucchini, tomatoes, shallot, and oregano in a bowl. Add salt and pepper to taste. Take 4 sheets of baking paper and arrange them on your working surface. Spoon the vegetable mixture in the center of each sheet.
2. Top with a fish fillet then wrap the paper well so it resembles a pocket. Place the wrapped fish in a baking tray and cook in

the preheated oven at 350 F/176 C for 15 minutes. Serve the fish warm and fresh.

Nutrition (for 100g):

149 Calories

2.8g Fat

5.2g Carbohydrates

25.2g Protein

696mg Sodium

237.   Creamy Smoked Salmon Pasta

Preparation Time: 5 minutes

Cooking Time: 35 minutes

Servings: 4

Ingredients

- 2 tbsps. olive oil
- 2 chopped garlic cloves
- 1 shallot, chopped
- 4 oz. or 113 g chopped salmon, smoked
- 1 c. green peas
- 1 c. heavy cream
- Salt and pepper
- 1 pinch chili flakes
- 8 oz. or 230 g penne pasta
- 6 c. water

Directions:

1. Place skillet on medium-high heat and add oil. Add the garlic and shallot. Cook for 5 minutes or until softened. Add peas, salt, pepper, and chili flakes. Cook for 10 minutes
2. Add the salmon, and continue cooking for 5-7 minutes more. Add heavy cream, reduce heat and cook for an extra 5 minutes.
3. In the meantime, place a pan with water and salt to your taste on high heat as soon as it boils, add penne pasta and cook for 8-10 minutes or until softened   Drain the pasta, add to the salmon sauce and serve

Nutrition (for 100g):

393 Calories

20.8g Fat

38g Carbohydrates

3g Protein

836mg Sodium

238. Slow Cooker Greek Chicken

Preparation Time 20 minutes

Cooking Time: 3 hours

Servings: 4

Ingredients

- 1 tablespoon extra-virgin olive oil
- 2 pounds boneless, chicken breasts
- ½ tsp kosher salt
- ¼ tsp black pepper
- 1 (12-ounce) jar roasted red peppers
- 1 cup Kalamata olives
- 1 medium red onion, cut into chunks
- 3 tablespoons red wine vinegar
- 1 tablespoon minced garlic
- 1 teaspoon honey
- 1 teaspoon dried oregano
- 1 teaspoon dried thyme
- ½ cup feta cheese (optional, for serving)
- Chopped fresh herbs: any mix of basil, parsley, or thyme (optional, for serving)

Directions

1. Brush slow cooker with nonstick cooking spray or olive oil. Cook the olive oil in a large skillet. Season both side of the chicken breasts. Once the oil is hot, add the chicken breasts and sear on both sides (about 3 minutes).
2. Once cooked, transfer it to the slow cooker. Add the red peppers, olives, and red onion to the chicken breasts. Try to place the vegetables around the chicken and not directly on top.
3. In a small bowl, mix together the vinegar, garlic, honey, oregano, and thyme. Once combined, pour it over the chicken. Cook

the chicken on low for 3 hours or until no longer pink in the middle. Serve with crumbled feta cheese and fresh herbs.

Nutrition (for 100g):

399 Calories

17g Fat

12g Carbohydrates

50g Protein

793mg Sodium

239. Chicken Gyros

Preparation Time 10 minutes

Cooking Time: 4 hours

Servings: 4

Ingredients

- 2 lbs. boneless chicken breasts or chicken tenders
- Juice of one lemon
- 3 cloves garlic
- 2 teaspoons red wine vinegar
- 2–3 tablespoons olive oil
- ½ cup Greek yogurt
- 2 teaspoons dried oregano
- 2–4 teaspoons Greek seasoning
- ½ small red onion, chopped
- 2 tablespoons dill weed
- Tzatziki Sauce
- 1 cup plain Greek yogurt
- 1 tablespoon dill weed
- 1 small English cucumber, chopped
- Pinch of salt and pepper
- 1 teaspoon onion powder
- Toppings: tomatoes, chopped cucumbers, chopped red onion, diced feta cheese, crumbled pita bread

Directions

1. Slice the chicken breasts into cubes and place in the slow cooker. Add the lemon juice, garlic, vinegar, olive oil, Greek yogurt, oregano, Greek seasoning, red

onion, and dill to the slow cooker and stir to make sure everything is well combined.

2. Cook on low for 5–6 hours or on high for 2–3 hours. In the meantime, incorporate all ingredients for the tzatziki sauce and stir. When well mixed, put in the refrigerator until the chicken is done.

3. When the chicken has finished cooking, serve with pita bread and any or all of the toppings listed above.

Nutrition (for 100g):

317 Calories

7.4g Fat

36.1g Carbohydrates

28.6g Protein

476mg Sodium

240. Slow Cooker Chicken Cassoulet

Preparation Time: 10 minutes

Cooking Time: 20 minutes

Servings: 16

Ingredients

- 1 cup dry navy beans, soaked
- 8 bone-in skinless chicken thighs
- 1 Polish sausage, cooked and chopped into bite-sized pieces (optional)
- 1¼ cup tomato juice
- 1 (28-ounce) can halved tomatoes
- 1 tbsp Worcestershire sauce
- 1 tsp instant beef or chicken bouillon granules
- ½ tsp dried basil
- ½ teaspoon dried oregano
- ½ teaspoon paprika
- ½ cup chopped celery
- ½ cup chopped carrot
- ½ cup chopped onion

Directions

1. Brush the slow cooker with olive oil or nonstick cooking spray. In a mixing bowl, stir together the tomato juice, tomatoes,

Worcestershire sauce, beef bouillon, basil, oregano, and paprika. Make sure the ingredients are well combined.

2. Place the chicken and sausage into the slow cooker and cover with the tomato juice mixture. Top with celery, carrot, and onion. Cook on low for 10–12 hours.

Nutrition (for 100g):

244 Calories

7g Fat

25g Carbohydrates

21g Protein

736mg Sodium

241. Slow Cooker Chicken Provencal

Preparation Time 5 minutes

Cooking Time: 8 hours

Servings: 4

Ingredients

- 4 (6-ounce) skinless bone-in chicken breast halves
- 2 teaspoons dried basil
- 1 teaspoon dried thyme
- 1/8 teaspoon salt
- 1/8 teaspoon freshly ground black pepper
- 1 yellow pepper, diced
- 1 red pepper, diced
- 1 (15.5-ounce) can cannellini beans
- 1 (14.5-ounce) can petite tomatoes with basil, garlic, and oregano, undrained

Directions

1. Brush the slow cooker with nonstick olive oil. Add all the ingredients to the slow cooker and stir to combine. Cook on low for 8 hours.

Nutrition (for 100g):

304 Calories

4.5g Fat

27.3g Carbohydrates

39.4g Protein

639mg Sodium

242.   Greek Style Turkey Roast

Preparation Time: 20 minutes

Cooking Time: 7 hours and 30 minutes

Servings: 8

Ingredients

- 1 (4-pound) boneless turkey breast, trimmed
- ½ cup chicken broth, divided
- 2 tablespoons fresh lemon juice
- 2 cups chopped onion
- ½ cup pitted Kalamata olives
- ½ cup oil-packed sun-dried tomatoes, thinly sliced
- 1 teaspoon Greek seasoning
- ½ teaspoon salt
- ¼ teaspoon fresh ground black pepper
- 3 tablespoons all-purpose flour (or whole wheat)

Directions

2. Brush the slow cooker with nonstick cooking spray or olive oil. Add the turkey, ¼ cup of the chicken broth, lemon juice, onion, olives, sun-dried tomatoes, Greek seasoning, salt and pepper to the slow cooker.
3. Cook on low for 7 hours. Scourge the flour into the remaining ¼ cup of chicken broth, then stir gently into the slow cooker. Cook for an additional 30 minutes.

Nutrition (for 100g):

341 Calories

19g Fat

12g Carbohydrates

36.4g Protein

639mg Sodium

243.   Garlic Chicken with Couscous

Preparation Time: 25 minutes

Cooking Time: 7 hours

Servings: 4

Ingredients

- 1 whole chicken, cut into pieces
- 1 tablespoon extra-virgin olive oil
- 6 cloves garlic, halved
- 1 cup dry white wine
- 1 cup couscous
- ½ teaspoon salt
- ½ teaspoon pepper
- 1 medium onion, thinly sliced
- 2 teaspoons dried thyme
- 1/3 cup whole wheat flour

Directions

1. Cook the olive oil in a heavy skillet. When skillet is hot, add the chicken to sear. Make sure the chicken pieces don't touch each other. Cook with the skin side down for about 3 minutes or until browned.
2. Brush your slow cooker with nonstick cooking spray or olive oil. Put the onion, garlic, and thyme into the slow cooker and sprinkle with salt and pepper. Stir in the chicken on top of the onions.
3. In a separate bowl, whisk the flour into the wine until there are no lumps, then pour over the chicken. Cook on low for 7 hours or until done. You can cook on high for 3 hours as well. Serve the chicken over the cooked couscous and spoon sauce over the top.

Nutrition (for 100g):

440 Calories

17.5g Fat

14g Carbohydrates

35.8g Protein

674mg Sodium

244. Chicken Karahi

Preparation Time: 5 minutes

Cooking Time: 5 hours

Servings: 4

Ingredients

- 2 lbs. chicken breasts or thighs
- ¼ cup olive oil
- 1 small can tomato paste
- 1 tablespoon butter
- 1 large onion, diced
- ½ cup plain Greek yogurt
- ½ cup water
- 2 tablespoons ginger in garlic paste
- 3 tablespoons fenugreek leaves
- 1 teaspoon ground coriander
- 1 medium tomato
- 1 teaspoon red chili
- 2 green chilies
- 1 teaspoon turmeric
- 1 tablespoon garam masala
- 1 teaspoon cumin powder
- 1 teaspoon sea salt
- ¼ teaspoon nutmeg

Directions

1. Brush the slow cooker with nonstick cooking spray. In a small bowl, thoroughly mix together all of the spices. Mix in the chicken to the slow cooker followed by the rest of the ingredients, including the spice mixture. Stir until everything is well mixed with the spices.
2. Cook on low for 4–5 hours. Serve with naan or Italian bread.

Nutrition (for 100g):

345 Calories

9.9g Fat

10g Carbohydrates

53.7g Protein

715mg Sodium

245. Chicken Cacciatore with Orzo

Preparation Time: 20 minutes

Cooking Time: 4 hours

Servings: 6

Ingredients

- 2 pounds skin-on chicken thighs
- 1 tablespoon olive oil
- 1 cup mushrooms, quartered
- 3 carrots, chopped
- 1 small jar Kalamata olives
- 2 (14-ounce) cans diced tomatoes
- 1 small can tomato paste
- 1 cup red wine
- 5 garlic cloves
- 1 cup orzo

Directions

1. In a large skillet, cook the olive oil. When the oil is heated, add the chicken, skin side down, and sear it. Make sure the pieces of chicken don't touch each other.
2. When the chicken is browned, add to the slow cooker along with all the ingredients except the orzo. Cook the chicken on low for 2 hours, then add the orzo and cook for an additional 2 hours. Serve with a crusty French bread.

Nutrition (for 100g):

424 Calories

16g Fat

10g Carbohydrates

11g Protein

845mg Sodium

Salad and sides Recipes

246. Peppers and Lentils Salad

Preparation Time: 10 minutes

Cooking Time: 0 minutes

Servings: 4

Size/ Portion: 2 cups

Ingredients:

- 14 ounces canned lentils
- 2 spring onions
- 1 red bell pepper
- 1 green bell pepper
- 1 tablespoon fresh lime juice
- 1/3 cup coriander
- 2 teaspoon balsamic vinegar

Directions:

1. In a salad bowl, combine the lentils with the onions, bell peppers, and the rest of the ingredients, toss and serve.

Nutrition:

200 Calories

2.45g Fat

5.6g Protein

247. Cashews and Red Cabbage Salad

Preparation Time: 10 minutes

Cooking Time: 0 minutes

 Servings: 4

Size/ Portion: 2 cups

Ingredients:

- 1-pound red cabbage, shredded
- 2 tablespoons coriander, chopped
- ½ cup cashews halved
- 2 tablespoons olive oil
- 1 tomato, cubed
- A pinch of salt and black pepper
- 1 tablespoon white vinegar

Directions:

1. Mix the cabbage with the coriander and the rest of the ingredients in a salad bowl, toss and serve cold.

Nutrition:

210 Calories

6.3g Fat

8g Protein

248. Tuscan Kale Salad with Anchovies

Preparation Time: 45 minutes

Cooking Time: 0 minute

Serving: 4

Size/ Portion: 2 cups

Ingredients:

- 1 large bunch Lacinato
- ¼ cup toasted pine nuts
- 1 cup Parmesan cheese
- ¼ cup extra-virgin olive oil
- 8 anchovy fillets
- 2 to 3 tablespoons lemon juice
- 2 teaspoons red pepper flakes (optional)

Direction:

1. Remove the rough center stems from the kale leaves and roughly tear each leaf into about 4-by-1-inch strips. Situate torn kale in a large bowl and add the pine nuts and cheese.

2. Blend the olive oil, anchovies, lemon juice, and red pepper flakes (if using). Drizzle over the salad and toss to coat well. Let sit at room temperature 30 minutes before serving, tossing again just prior to serving.

Nutrition:

337 Calories

25g Fat

16g Protein

249. Apples and Pomegranate Salad

Preparation Time: 10 minutes

Cooking Time: 0 minutes

Servings: 4

Size/ Portion: 2 cups

Ingredients:

- 3 big apples, cored and cubed
- 1 cup pomegranate seeds
- 3 cups baby arugula
- 1 cup walnuts, chopped
- 1 tablespoon olive oil
- 1 teaspoon white sesame seeds
- 2 tablespoons apple cider vinegar

Directions:

1. Mix the apples with the arugula and the rest of the ingredients in a bowl, toss and serve cold.

Nutrition:

160 Calories

4.3g Fat

10g Protein

250. Cranberry Bulgur Mix

Preparation Time: 10 minutes

Cooking Time: 0 minutes

Servings: 4

Size/ Portion: 2 cups

Ingredients:

- 1 and ½ cups hot water
- 1 cup bulgur
- Juice of ½ lemon
- 4 tablespoons cilantro, chopped
- ½ cup cranberries
- 1 and ½ teaspoons curry powder
- ¼ cup green onions
- ½ cup red bell peppers
- ½ cup carrots, grated
- 1 tablespoon olive oil

Directions:

1. Put bulgur into a bowl, add the water, stir, cover, leave aside for 10 minutes, fluff with a fork, and transfer to a bowl. Add the rest of the ingredients, toss, and serve cold.

Nutrition:

300 Calories

6.4g Fat

13g Protein

251. Chickpeas, Corn and Black Beans Salad

Preparation Time: 10 minutes

Cooking Time: 0 minutes

Servings: 4

Size/ Portion: 2 cups

Ingredients:

- 1 and ½ cups canned black beans

- ½ teaspoon garlic powder

- 2 teaspoons chili powder

- 1 and ½ cups canned chickpeas

- 1 cup baby spinach

- 1 avocado, pitted, peeled, and chopped

- 1 cup corn kernels, chopped

- 2 tablespoons lemon juice

- 1 tablespoon olive oil

- 1 tablespoon apple cider vinegar

- 1 teaspoon chives, chopped

Directions:

1. Mix the black beans with the garlic powder, chili powder, and the rest of the ingredients in a bowl, toss and serve cold.

Nutrition:

300 Calories

13.4g Fat

13g Protein

252.   Olives and Lentils Salad

Preparation Time: 10 minutes

Cooking Time: 0 minutes

Servings: 2

Size/ Portion: 2 cups

Ingredients:

- 1/3 cup canned green lentils

- 1 tablespoon olive oil

- 2 cups baby spinach

- 1 cup black olives

- 2 tablespoons sunflower seeds

- 1 tablespoon Dijon mustard

- 2 tablespoons balsamic vinegar

- 2 tablespoons olive oil

Directions:

1. Mix the lentils with the spinach, olives, and the rest of the ingredients in a salad bowl, toss and serve cold.

Nutrition:

279 Calories

6.5g Fat

12g Protein

253.   Lime Spinach and Chickpeas Salad

Preparation Time: 10 minutes

Cooking Time: 0 minutes

Servings: 4

Size/ Portion: 2 cups

Ingredients:

- 16 ounces canned chickpeas

- 2 cups baby spinach leaves

- ½ tablespoon lime juice

- 2 tablespoons olive oil

- 1 teaspoon cumin, ground

- ½ teaspoon chili flakes

Directions:

1. Mix the chickpeas with the spinach and the rest of the ingredients in a large bowl, toss and serve cold.

Nutrition:

240 calories

8.2g fat

12g protein

254.   Minty Olives and Tomatoes Salad

Preparation Time: 10 minutes

Cooking Time: 0 minutes

Servings: 4

Size/ Portion: 2 cups

Ingredients:

- 1 cup kalamata olives
- 1 cup black olives
- 1 cup cherry tomatoes
- 4 tomatoes
- 1 red onion, chopped
- 2 tablespoons oregano, chopped
- 1 tablespoon mint, chopped
- 2 tablespoons balsamic vinegar
- ¼ cup olive oil
- 2 teaspoons Italian herbs, dried

Directions:

1. In a salad bowl, mix the olives with the tomatoes and the rest of the ingredients, toss, and serve cold.

Nutrition:

190 Calories

8.1g Fat

4.6g Protein

255. Beans and Cucumber Salad

Preparation Time: 10 minutes

Cooking Time: 0 minutes

Servings: 4

Size/ Portion: 2 cups

Ingredients:

- 15 g canned great northern beans
- 2 tablespoons olive oil
- ½ cup baby arugula
- 1 cup cucumber
- 1 tablespoon parsley
- 2 tomatoes, cubed
- 2 tablespoon balsamic vinegar

Directions:

1. Mix the beans with the cucumber and the rest of the ingredients in a large bowl, toss and serve cold.

Nutrition:

233 calories

9g fat

8g protein

256. Tomato and Avocado Salad

Preparation Time: 10 minutes

Cooking Time: 0 minutes

Servings: 4

Size/ Portion: 2 cups

Ingredients:

- 1-pound cherry tomatoes
- 2 avocados
- 1 sweet onion, chopped
- 2 tablespoons lemon juice
- 1 and ½ tablespoons olive oil
- Handful basil, chopped

Directions:

1. Mix the tomatoes with the avocados and the rest of the ingredients in a serving bowl, toss and serve right away.

Nutrition:

148 Calories

7.8g Fat

5.5g Protein

257. Arugula Salad

Preparation Time: 5 minutes

Cooking Time: 0 minutes

Servings: 4

Size/ Portion: 2 cups

Ingredients:

- Arugula leaves (4 cups)
- Cherry tomatoes (1 cup)
- Pine nuts (.25 cup)
- Rice vinegar (1 tbsp.)
- Olive/grapeseed oil (2 tbsp.)
- Grated parmesan cheese (.25 cup)
- Black pepper & salt (as desired)
- Large sliced avocado (1)

Directions:

1. Peel and slice the avocado. Rinse and dry the arugula leaves, grate the cheese, and slice the cherry tomatoes into halves.

2. Combine the arugula, pine nuts, tomatoes, oil, vinegar, salt, pepper, and cheese.

3. Toss the salad to mix and portion it onto plates with the avocado slices to serve.

Nutrition:

257 Calories

23g Fats

6.1g Protein

258. Chickpea Salad

Preparation Time: 15 minutes

Cooking Time: 0 minutes

Servings: 4

Size/ Portion: 2 cups

Ingredients:

- Cooked chickpeas (15 g)
- Diced Roma tomato (1)
- Diced green medium bell pepper (half of 1)
- Fresh parsley (1 tbsp.)
- Small white onion (1)
- Minced garlic (.5 tsp.)
- Lemon (1 juiced)

Directions:

1. Chop the tomato, green pepper, and onion. Mince the garlic. Combine each of the fixings into a salad bowl and toss well.

2. Cover the salad to chill for at least 15 minutes in the fridge. Serve when ready.

Nutrition:

163 Calories

7g Fats

4g Protein

259. Chopped Israeli Mediterranean Pasta Salad

Preparation Time: 15 minutes

Cooking Time: 2 minutes

Servings: 8

Size/ Portion: 2 cups

Ingredients:

- Small bow tie or other small pasta (.5 lb.)
- 1/3 cup Cucumber
- 1/3 cup Radish
- 1/3 cup Tomato
- 1/3 cup Yellow bell pepper
- 1/3 cup Orange bell pepper

- 1/3 cup Black olives
- 1/3 cup Green olives
- 1/3 cup Red onions
- 1/3 cup Pepperoncini
- 1/3 cup Feta cheese
- 1/3 cup Fresh thyme leaves
- Dried oregano (1 tsp.)

Dressing:

- 0.25 cup + more, olive oil
- juice of 1 lemon

Directions:

1. Slice the green olives into halves. Dice the feta and pepperoncini. Finely dice the remainder of the veggies.

2. Prepare a pot of water with the salt, and simmer the pasta until its al dente (checking at two minutes under the listed time). Rinse and drain in cold water.

3. Combine a small amount of oil with the pasta. Add the salt, pepper, oregano, thyme, and veggies. Pour in the rest of the oil, lemon juice, and mix and fold in the grated feta.

4. Pop it into the fridge within two hours, best if overnight. Taste test and adjust the seasonings to your liking; add fresh thyme.

Nutrition:

65 Calories

5.6g Fats

0.8g Protein

260. Greek Pasta Salad

Preparation Time: 5 minutes

Cooking Time: 11 minutes

Servings: 4

Size/ Portion: 2 cups

Ingredients:

- Penne pasta (1 cup)
- Lemon juice (1.5 tsp.)
- Red wine vinegar (2 tbsp.)
- Garlic (1 clove)
- Dried oregano (1 tsp.)
- Black pepper and sea salt (as desired)
- Olive oil (.33 cup)
- Halved cherry tomatoes (5)
- Red onion (half of 1 small)
- Green & red bell pepper (half of 1 - each)
- Cucumber (¼ of 1)
- Black olives (.25 cup)
- Crumbled feta cheese (.25 cup)

Directions:

1. Slice the cucumber and olives. Chop/dice the onion, peppers, and garlic. Slice the tomatoes into halves.

2. Arrange a large pot with water and salt using the high-temperature setting. Once it's boiling, add the pasta and cook for 11 minutes Rinse it using cold water and drain in a colander.

3. Whisk the oil, juice, salt, pepper, vinegar, oregano, and garlic. Combine the cucumber, cheese, olives, peppers, pasta, onions, and tomatoes in a large salad dish.

4. Add the vinaigrette over the pasta and toss. Chill in the fridge (covered) for about three hours and serve as desired.

Nutrition:

307 Calories

23.6g Fat

5.4g Protein

Breakfast (Salad Recipes)

261. Feta Beet Salad

Preparation Time: 16 minutes

Cooking Time: 0 minute

Serving: 4

Size/ Portion: 2 cups

Ingredients:

- 6 Red Beets, Cooked & Peeled
- 3 Ounces Feta Cheese, Cubed
- 2 Tablespoons Olive Oil
- 2 Tablespoons Balsamic Vinegar

Directions:

1. Combine everything together, and then serve.

Nutrition:

230 Calories

7.3g Protein

12g Fat

262. Zucchini Pasta

Preparation Time: 9 minutes

Cooking Time: 32 minutes

Serving: 4

Size/ Portion: 2 ounces

Ingredients:

- 3 tablespoons olive oil
- 2 cloves garlic, minced
- 3 zucchinis, large & diced
- sea salt & black pepper to taste
- ½ cup milk, 2%
- ¼ teaspoon nutmeg
- 1 tablespoon lemon juice, fresh
- ½ cup parmesan, grated
- 8 ounces uncooked farfalle pasta

Directions:

1. Get out a skillet and place it over medium heat, and then heat up the oil. Add in your garlic and cook for a minute. Stir often so that it doesn't burn. Add in your salt, pepper and zucchini. Stir well, and cook covered for fifteen minutes. During this time, you'll want to stir the mixture twice.

2. Get out a microwave safe bowl, and heat the milk for thirty seconds. Stir in your nutmeg, and then pour it into the skillet. Cook uncovered for five minutes. Stir occasionally to keep from burning.

3. Get out a stockpot and cook your pasta per package instructions. Drain the pasta, and then save two tablespoons of pasta water.

4. Stir everything together, and add in the cheese and lemon juice and pasta water.

Nutrition

410 Calories

15g Protein

17g Fat

263. Watermelon Salad

Preparation Time: 18 minutes

Cooking Time: 0 minute

Serving: 6

Size/ Portion: 2 cups

Ingredients:

- ¼ teaspoon sea salt
- ¼ teaspoon black pepper
- 1 tablespoon balsamic vinegar

- 1 cantaloupe, quartered & seeded
- 12 watermelon, small & seedless
- 2 cups mozzarella balls, fresh
- 1/3 cup basil, fresh & torn
- 2 tablespoons olive oil

Directions:

1. Scoop out balls of cantaloupe, and the put them in a colander over bowl.
2. With a melon baller slice the watermelon.
3. Allow your fruit to drain for ten minutes, and then refrigerate the juice.
4. Wipe the bowl dry, and then place your fruit in it.
5. Stir in basil, oil, vinegar, mozzarella and tomatoes before seasoning.
6. Mix well and serve.

Nutrition:

218 Calories

10g Protein

13g Fat

264.   Orange Celery Salad

Preparation Time: 16 minutes

Cooking Time: 0 minute

Serving: 6

Size/ Portion: 2 cups

Ingredients:

- 1 tablespoon lemon juice, fresh
- ¼ teaspoon sea salt, fine
- ¼ teaspoon black pepper
- 1 tablespoon olive brine
- 1 tablespoon olive oil
- ¼ cup red onion, sliced

- ½ cup green olives
- 2 oranges, peeled & sliced
- 3 celery stalks, sliced diagonally in ½ inch slices

Directions:

1. Put your oranges, olives, onion and celery in a shallow bowl.
2. Stir oil, olive brine and lemon juice, pour this over your salad.
3. Season with salt and pepper before serving.

Nutrition:

65 Calories

2g Protein

0.2g Fat

265.   Roasted Broccoli Salad

Preparation Time: 9 minutes

Cooking Time: 17 minutes

Serving: 4

Size/ portion: 2 cups

Ingredients:

- 1 lb. broccoli
- 3 tablespoons olive oil, divided
- 1-pint cherry tomatoes
- 1 ½ teaspoons honey
- 3 cups cubed bread, whole grain
- 1 tablespoon balsamic vinegar
- ½ teaspoon black pepper
- ¼ teaspoon sea salt, fine
- grated parmesan for serving

Directions:

1. Set oven to 450, and then place rimmed baking sheet.

2. Drizzle your broccoli with a tablespoon of oil, and toss to coat.

3. Take out from oven, and spoon the broccoli. Leave oil at bottom of the bowl and add in your tomatoes, toss to coat, then mix tomatoes with a tablespoon of honey. Place on the same baking sheet.

4. Roast for fifteen minutes, and stir halfway through your cooking time.

5. Add in your bread, and then roast for three more minutes.

6. Whisk two tablespoons of oil, vinegar, and remaining honey. Season. Pour this over your broccoli mix to serve.

Nutrition:

226 Calories

7g Protein

12g Fat

266. Tomato Salad

Preparation Time: 22 minutes

Cooking Time: 0 minute

Serving: 4

Size/ portion: 2 cups

Ingredients:

- 1 cucumber, sliced

- ¼ cup sun dried tomatoes, chopped

- 1 lb. tomatoes, cubed

- ½ cup black olives

- 1 red onion, sliced

- 1 tablespoon balsamic vinegar

- ¼ cup parsley, fresh & chopped

- 2 tablespoons olive oil

Directions:

1. Get out a bowl and combine all of your vegetables together. To make your dressing mix all your seasoning, olive oil and vinegar.

2. Toss with your salad and serve fresh.

Nutrition

126 Calories

2.1g Protein

9.2g Fat

267. Tahini Spinach

Preparation Time: 11 minutes

Cooking Time: 6 minutes

Serving: 3

Size/ Portion: 2 cups

Ingredients:

- 10 spinach, chopped

- ½ cup water

- 1 tablespoon tahini

- 2 cloves garlic, minced

- ¼ teaspoon cumin

- ¼ teaspoon paprika

- ¼ teaspoon cayenne pepper

- 1/3 cup red wine vinegar

Direction:

1. Add your spinach and water to the saucepan, and then boil it on high heat. Once boiling reduce to low, and cover. Allow it to cook on simmer for five minutes.

2. Add in your garlic, cumin, cayenne, red wine vinegar, paprika and tahini. Whisk well, and season with salt and pepper.

3. Drain your spinach and top with tahini sauce to serve.

Nutrition:

69 Calories

5g Protein

3g Fat

268. Pilaf with Cream Cheese

Preparation Time: 11 minutes

Cooking Time: 34 minutes

Serving: 6

Size/ Portion: 2 cups

Ingredients:

- 2 cups yellow long grain rice, parboiled
- 1 cup onion
- 4 green onions
- 3 tablespoons butter
- 3 tablespoons vegetable broth
- 2 teaspoons cayenne pepper
- 1 teaspoon paprika
- ½ teaspoon cloves, minced
- 2 tablespoons mint leaves
- 1 bunch fresh mint leaves to garnish
- 1 tablespoons olive oil

Cheese Cream:

- 3 tablespoons olive oil
- sea salt & black pepper to taste
- 9 ounces cream cheese

Directions:

1. Start by heating your oven to 360, and then get out a pan. Heat your butter and olive oil together, and cook your onions and spring onions for two minutes.

2. Add in your salt, pepper, paprika, cloves, vegetable broth, rice and remaining seasoning. S

3. Sauté for three minutes.

4. Wrap with foil, and bake for another half hour. Allow it to cool.

5. Mix in the cream cheese, cheese, olive oil, salt and pepper. Serve your pilaf garnished with fresh mint leaves.

Nutrition:

364 Calories

5g Protein

30g Fat

269. Easy Spaghetti Squash

Preparation Time: 13 minutes

Cooking Time: 45 minutes

Serving: 6

Size/ Portion: 2 ounces

Ingredients:

- 2 spring onions, chopped fine
- 3 cloves garlic, minced
- 1 zucchini, diced
- 1 red bell pepper, diced
- 1 tablespoon Italian seasoning
- 1 tomato, small & chopped fine
- 1 tablespoons parsley, fresh & chopped
- pinch lemon pepper
- dash sea salt, fine
- 4 ounces feta cheese, crumbled
- 3 Italian sausage links, casing removed
- 2 tablespoons olive oil
- 1 spaghetti sauce, halved lengthwise

Directions:

1. Prep oven to 350, and get out a large baking sheet. Coat it with cooking spray, and then put your squash on it with the cut side down.

2. Bake at 350 for forty-five minutes. It should be tender.

3. Turn the squash over, and bake for five more minutes. Scrape the strands into a larger bowl.

4. Cook tablespoon of olive oil in a skillet, and then add in your Italian sausage. Cook at eight minutes before removing it and placing it in a bowl.

5. Add another tablespoon of olive oil to the skillet and cook your garlic and onions until softened. This will take five minutes. Throw in your Italian seasoning, red peppers and zucchini. Cook for another five minutes. Your vegetables should be softened.

6. Mix in your feta cheese and squash, cooking until the cheese has melted.

7. Stir in your sausage, and then season with lemon pepper and salt. Serve with parsley and tomato.

Nutrition:

423 Calories

18g Protein

30g Fat

270.   Roasted Eggplant Salad

Preparation Time: 14 minutes

Cooking Time: 36 minutes

Serving: 6

Size/ Portion: 2 cups

Ingredients:

- 1 red onion, sliced

- 2 tablespoons parsley

- 1 teaspoon thyme

- 2 cups cherry tomatoes

- 1 teaspoon oregano

- 3 tablespoons olive oil

- 1 teaspoon basil

- 3 eggplants, peeled & cubed

Directions:

1. Start by heating your oven to 350.

2. Season your eggplant with basil, salt, pepper, oregano, thyme and olive oil.

3. Arrange it on a baking tray, and bake for a half hour.

4. Toss with your remaining ingredients before serving.

Nutrition:

148 Calories

3.5g Protein

7.7g Fat

271.   Penne with Tahini Sauce

Preparation Time: 16 minutes

Cooking Time: 22 minutes

Serving: 8

Size/ Portion: 2 ounces

Ingredients:

- 1/3 cup water

- 1 cup yogurt, plain

- 1/8 cup lemon juice

- 3 tablespoons tahini

- 3 cloves garlic

- 1 onion, chopped

- ¼ cup olive oil

- 2 portobello mushrooms, large & sliced
- ½ red bell pepper, diced
- 16 ounces penne pasta
- ½ cup parsley, fresh & chopped

Directions:

1. Start by getting out a pot and bring a pot of salted water to a boil. Cook your pasta al dente per package instructions.

2. Mix your lemon juice and tahini together, and then place it in a food processor. Process with garlic, water and yogurt.

3. Situate pan over medium heat. Heat up your oil, and cook your onions until soft.

4. Add in your mushroom and continue to cook until softened.

5. Add in your bell pepper, and cook until crispy.

6. Drain your pasta, and then toss with your tahini sauce, top with parsley and pepper and serve with vegetables.

Nutrition:

332 Calories

11g Proteins

12g Fat

272.   Asparagus Pasta

Preparation Time: 8 minutes

Cooking Time: 33 minutes

Serving: 6

Size/ Portion: 2 ounces

Ingredients:

- 8 ounces farfalle pasta, uncooked
- 1 ½ cups asparagus
- 1-pint grape tomatoes, halved
- 2 tablespoons olive oil

- 2 cups mozzarella, fresh & drained
- 1/3 cup basil leaves, fresh & torn
- 2 tablespoons balsamic vinegar

Directions:

1. Start by heating the oven to 400, and then get out a stockpot. Cook your pasta per package instructions, and reserve ¼ cup of pasta water.

2. Get out a bowl and toss the tomatoes, oil, asparagus, and season with salt and pepper. Spread this mixture on a baking sheet, and bake for fifteen minutes. Stir twice in this time.

3. Remove your vegetables from the oven, and then add the cooked pasta to your baking sheet. Mix with a few tablespoons of pasta water so that your sauce becomes smoother.

4. Mix in your basil and mozzarella, drizzling with balsamic vinegar. Serve warm.

Nutrition:

307 Calories

18g Protein

14g Fat

273.   Feta & Spinach Pita Bake

Time: 11 minutes

Cooking Time: 36 minutes

Serving: 6

Size/ Portion: 2 ounces

Ingredients:

- 2 roma tomatoes
- 6 whole wheat pita bread
- 1 jar sun dried tomato pesto
- 4 mushrooms, fresh & sliced
- 1 bunch spinach

- 2 tablespoons parmesan cheese

- 3 tablespoons olive oil

- ½ cup feta cheese

Directions:

1. Start by heating the oven to 350, and get to your pita bread. Spread the tomato pesto on the side of each one. Put them in a baking pan with the tomato side up.

2. Top with tomatoes, spinach, mushrooms, parmesan and feta. Drizzle with olive oil and season with pepper.

3. Bake for twelve minutes, and then serve cut into quarters.

Nutrition:

350 Calories

12g Protein

17g Fat

Eggs Recipes

274. Denver Fried Omelet

Preparation Time: 10 minutes

Cooking Time: 30 minutes

Servings: 4

Ingredients:

- 2 tablespoons butter
- 1/2 onion, minced meat
- 1/2 green pepper, minced
- 1 cup chopped cooked ham
- 8 eggs
- 1/4 cup of milk
- 1/2 cup grated cheddar cheese and ground black pepper to taste

Directions:

1. Preheat the oven to 200 degrees C (400 degrees F). Grease a round baking dish of 10 inches.
2. Melt the butter over medium heat; cook and stir onion and pepper until soft, about 5 minutes. Stir in the ham and keep cooking until everything is hot for 5 minutes.
3. Whip the eggs and milk in a large bowl. Stir in the mixture of cheddar cheese and ham; Season with salt and black pepper. Pour the mixture in a baking dish. Bake in the oven, about 25 minutes. Serve hot.

Nutrition (for 100g):

345 Calories

26.8g Fat

3.6g Carbohydrates

22.4g Protein

712 mg Sodium

275. Sausage Pan

Preparation Time: 25 minutes

Cooking Time: 1 hour

Servings: 12

Ingredients:

- 1-pound Sage Breakfast Sausage,
- 3 cups grated potatoes, drained and squeezed
- 1/4 cup melted butter,
- 12 oz soft grated Cheddar cheese
- 1/2 cup onion, grated
- 1 (16 oz) small cottage cheese container
- 6 giant eggs

Directions:

1. Set up the oven to 190 ° C. Grease a 9 x 13-inch square oven dish lightly.
2. Place the sausage in a big deep-frying pan. Bake over medium heat until smooth. Drain, crumble, and reserve.
3. Mix the grated potatoes and butter in the prepared baking dish. Cover the bottom and sides of the dish with the mixture. Combine in a bowl sausage, cheddar, onion, cottage cheese, and eggs. Pour over the potato mixture. Let it bake.
4. Allow cooling for 5 minutes before serving.

Nutrition (for 100g):

355 Calories

26.3g Fat

7.9g Carbohydrates

21.6g Protein

755mg Sodium.

276. Grilled Marinated Shrimp

Preparation Time: 30 minutes

Cooking Time: 1 hour

Servings: 6

Ingredients:

- 1 cup olive oil,
- 1/4 cup chopped fresh parsley
- 1 lemon, juiced,
- 3 cloves of garlic, finely chopped

- 1 tablespoon tomato puree
- 2 teaspoons dried oregano,
- 1 teaspoon salt
- 2 tablespoons hot pepper sauce
- 1 teaspoon ground black pepper,
- 2 pounds of shrimp, peeled and stripped of tails

Directions:

1. Combine olive oil, parsley, lemon juice, hot sauce, garlic, tomato puree, oregano, salt, and black pepper in a bowl. Reserve a small amount to string later. Fill the large, resealable plastic bag with marinade and shrimp. Close and let it chill for 2 hours.
2. Preheat the grill on medium heat. Thread shrimp on skewers, poke once at the tail, and once at the head. Discard the marinade.
3. Lightly oil the grill. Cook the prawns for 5 minutes on each side or until they are opaque, often baste with the reserved marinade.

Nutrition (for 100g):

447 Calories

37.5g Fat

3.7g Carbohydrates

25.3g Protein

800mg Sodium

277. Sausage Egg Casserole

Preparation Time: 20 minutes

Cooking Time: 1 hour 10 minutes

Servings: 12

Ingredients:

- 3/4-pound finely chopped pork sausage
- 1 tablespoon butter
- 4 green onions, minced meat
- 1/2 pound of fresh mushrooms
- 10 eggs, beaten
- 1 container (16 grams) low-fat cottage cheese

- 1 pound of Monterey Jack Cheese, grated
- 2 cans of a green pepper diced, drained
- 1 cup flour, 1 teaspoon baking powder
- 1/2 teaspoon salt
- 1/3 cup melted butter

Directions:

1. Put sausage in a deep-frying pan. Bake over medium heat until smooth. Drain and set aside. Melt the butter in a pan, cook and stir the green onions and mushrooms until they are soft.
2. Combine eggs, cottage cheese, Monterey Jack cheese, and peppers in a large bowl. Stir in sausages, green onions, and mushrooms. Cover and spend the night in the fridge.
3. Setup the oven to 175 ° C (350 ° F). Grease a 9 x 13-inch light baking dish.
4. Sift the flour, baking powder, and salt into a bowl. Stir in the melted butter. Incorporate flour mixture into the egg mixture. Pour into the prepared baking dish. Bake until lightly browned. Let stand for 10 minutes before serving.

Nutrition (for 100g):

408 Calories

28.7g Fat

12.4g Carbohydrates

25.2g Protein

1095mg Sodium

278. Baked Omelet Squares

Preparation Time: 15 Minutes

Cooking Time: 30 minutes

Servings: 8

Ingredients:

- 1/4 cup butter
- 1 small onion, minced meat
- 1 1/2 cups grated cheddar cheese
- 1 can of sliced mushrooms

- 1 can slice black olives cooked ham (optional)
- sliced jalapeno peppers (optional)
- 12 eggs, scrambled eggs
- 1/2 cup of milk
- salt and pepper, to taste

Directions:

1. Prepare the oven to 205 ° C (400 ° F). Grease a 9 x 13-inch baking dish.
2. Cook the butter in a frying pan over medium heat and cook the onion until done.
3. Lay out the Cheddar cheese on the bottom of the prepared baking dish. Layer with mushrooms, olives, fried onion, ham, and jalapeno peppers. Stir the eggs in a bowl with milk, salt, and pepper. Pour the egg mixture over the ingredients, but do not mix.
4. Bake in the uncovered and preheated oven, until no more liquid flows in the middle and is light brown above. Allow to cool a little, then cut it into squares and serve.

Nutrition (for 100g):

344 Calories

27.3g Fat

7.2g Carbohydrates

17.9g Protein

1087mg Sodium

279. Hard-Boiled Egg

Preparation Time: 5 minutes

Cooking Time: 15 minutes

Servings: 8

Ingredients:

- 1 tablespoon of salt
- 1/4 cup distilled white vinegar
- 6 cups of water
- 8 eggs

Directions:

1. Place the salt, vinegar, and water in a large saucepan and bring to a boil over high heat. Stir in the eggs one by one, and be careful not to split them. Lower the heat and cook over low heat and cook for 14 minutes.
2. Pull out the eggs from the hot water and place them in a container filled with ice water or cold water. Cool completely, approximately 15 minutes.

Nutrition (for 100g):

72 Calories

5g Fat

0.4g Carbohydrates

6.3g Protein

947 mg Sodium

280. Mushrooms with a Soy Sauce Glaze

Preparation Time: 5 minutes

Cooking Time: 10 minutes

Servings: 2

Ingredients:

- 2 tablespoons butter
- 1(8 ounces) package sliced white mushrooms
- 2 cloves garlic, minced
- 2 teaspoons soy sauce
- ground black pepper to taste

Directions:

1. Cook the butter in a frying pan over medium heat; stir in the mushrooms; cook and stir until the mushrooms are soft and released about 5 minutes. Stir in the garlic; keep cooking and stir for 1 minute. Pour the soy sauce; cook the mushrooms in the soy sauce until the liquid has evaporated, about 4 minutes.

Nutrition (for 100g):

135 Calories

11.9g Fat

5.4g Carbohydrates

4.2g Protein

387mg Sodium

281.   Pepperoni Eggs

Preparation Time: 10 minutes

Cooking Time: 20 minutes

Servings: 2

Ingredients:

- 1 cup of egg substitute
- 1 egg
- 3 green onions, minced meat
- 8 slices of pepperoni, diced
- 1/2 teaspoon of garlic powder
- 1 teaspoon melted butter
- 1/4 cup grated Romano cheese
- salt and ground black pepper to taste

Directions:

2. Combine the egg substitute, the egg, the green onions, the pepperoni slices, and the garlic powder in a bowl.
3. Cook the butter in a non-stick frying pan over low heat; Add the egg mixture, seal the pan and cook 10 to 15 minutes. Sprinkle Romano's eggs and season with salt and pepper.

Nutrition (for 100g):

266 Calories

16.2g Fat

3.7g Carbohydrates

25.3g Protein

586mg Sodium

282.   Egg Cupcakes

Preparation Time: 15 minutes

Cooking Time: 20 minutes

Servings: 6

Ingredients:

- 1 pack of bacon (12 ounces)
- 6 eggs
- 2 tablespoons of milk
- 1/4 teaspoon salt
- 1/4 teaspoon ground black pepper
- 1 c. Melted butter
- 1/4 teaspoon. Dried parsley
- 1/2 cup ham
- 1/4 cup mozzarella cheese
- 6 slices gouda

Directions:

1. Prepare the oven to 175 ° C (350 ° F). Cook bacon over medium heat, until it starts to brown. Dry the bacon slices with kitchen paper.
2. Situate the slices of bacon in the 6 cups of the non-stick muffin pan. Slice the remaining bacon and put it at the bottom of each cup.
3. Mix eggs, milk, butter, parsley, salt, and pepper. Add in the ham and mozzarella cheese.
4. Fill the cups with the egg mixture; garnish with Gouda cheese.
5. Bake in the preheated oven until Gouda cheese is melted and the eggs are tender about 15 minutes.

Nutrition (for 100g):

310 Calories

22.9g Fat

2.1g Carbohydrates

23.1g Protein

988mg Sodium.

283.   Dinosaur Eggs

Preparation Time: 20 minutes

Cooking Time: 15 minutes

Servings: 4

Ingredients:

- Mustard sauce:
- 1/4 cup coarse mustard
- 1/4 cup Greek yogurt
- 1 teaspoon garlic powder
- 1 pinch of cayenne pepper
- Eggs:
- 2 beaten eggs
- 2 cups of mashed potato flakes
- 4 boiled eggs, peeled
- 1 can (15 oz) HORMEL® Mary Kitchen® minced beef finely chopped can
- 2 liters of vegetable oil for frying

Directions:

1. Combine the old-fashioned mustard, Greek yogurt, garlic powder, and cayenne pepper in a small bowl until smooth.
2. Transfer the 2 beaten eggs in a shallow dish; place the potato flakes in a separate shallow dish.
3. Divide the minced meat into 4 Servings. Form salted beef around each egg until it is completely wrapped.
4. Soak the wrapped eggs in the beaten egg and brush with mashed potatoes until they are covered.
5. Fill the oil in a large saucepan and heat at 190 ° C (375 ° F).
6. Put 2 eggs in the hot oil and bake for 3 to 5 minutes until brown. Remove with a drop of spoon and place on a plate lined with kitchen paper. Repeat this with the remaining 2 eggs.
7. Cut lengthwise and serve with a mustard sauce.

Nutrition (for 100g):

784 Calories

63.2g Fat

34g Carbohydrates

19.9g Protein

702mg Sodium

284.   **Dill and Tomato Frittata**

Preparation Time: 10 minutes

Cooking Time: 35 minutes

Servings: 6

Ingredients:

- Pepper and salt to taste
- 1 teaspoon red pepper flakes
- 2 garlic cloves, minced
- ½ cup crumbled goat cheese – optional
- 2 tablespoon fresh chives, chopped
- 2 tablespoon fresh dill, chopped
- 4 tomatoes, diced
- 8 eggs, whisked
- 1 teaspoon coconut oil

Directions:

1. Grease a 9-inch round baking pan and preheat oven to 325oF.
2. In a large bowl, mix well all ingredients and pour into prepped pan.
3. Lay into the oven and bake until middle is cooked through around 30-35 minutes.
4. Remove from oven and garnish with more chives and dill.

Nutrition (for 100g):

149 Calories

10.28g Fat

9.93g Carbohydrates

13.26g Protein

523mg Sodium

285.   **Paleo Almond Banana Pancakes**

Preparation Time: 10 minutes

Cooking Time: 10 minutes

Servings: 3

Ingredients:

- ¼ cup almond flour
- ½ teaspoon ground cinnamon
- 3 eggs

- 1 banana, mashed
- 1 tablespoon almond butter
- 1 teaspoon vanilla extract
- 1 teaspoon olive oil
- Sliced banana to serve

Directions:

1. Whip eggs in a bowl until fluffy. In another bowl, mash the banana using a fork and add to the egg mixture. Add the vanilla, almond butter, cinnamon and almond flour. Mix into a smooth batter. Heat the olive oil in a skillet. Add one spoonful of the batter and fry them on both sides.
2. Keep doing these steps until you are done with all the batter.
3. Add some sliced banana on top before serving.

Nutrition (for 100g):

306 Calories

26g Fat

3.6g Carbohydrates

14.4g Protein

588mg Sodium

286.   Zucchini with Egg

Preparation Time: 5 minutes

Cooking Time: 10 minutes

Servings: 2

Ingredients:

- 1 1/2 tablespoons olive oil
- 2 large zucchinis, cut into large chunks
- salt and ground black pepper to taste
- 2 large eggs
- 1 teaspoon water, or as desired

Directions:

1. Cook the oil in a frying pan over medium heat; sauté zucchini until soft, about 10 minutes. Season the zucchini well.

2. Lash the eggs using a fork in a bowl. Pour in water and beat until everything is well mixed. Pour the eggs over the zucchini; boil and stir until scrambled eggs and no more flowing, about 5 minutes. Season well the zucchini and eggs.

Nutrition (for 100g):

213 Calories

15.7g Fat

11.2g Carbohydrates

10.2g Protein

180mg Sodium

287.   Cheesy Amish Breakfast Casserole

Preparation Time: 10 minutes

Cooking Time: 50 minutes

Servings: 12

Ingredients:

- 1-pound sliced bacon, diced,
- 1 sweet onion, minced meat
- 4 cups grated and frozen potatoes, thawed
- 9 lightly beaten eggs
- 2 cups of grated cheddar cheese
- 1 1/2 cup of cottage cheese
- 1 1/4 cups of grated Swiss cheese

Directions:

1. Preheat the oven to 175 ° C (350 ° F). Grease a 9 x 13-inch baking dish.
2. Warm up large frying pan over medium heat; cook and stir the bacon and onion until the bacon is evenly browned about 10 minutes. Drain. Stir in potatoes, eggs, cheddar cheese, cottage cheese, and Swiss cheese. Fill the mixture into a prepared baking dish.
3. Bake in the oven until the eggs are cooked and the cheese is melted 45 to 50 minutes. Set aside for 10 minutes before cutting and serving.

Nutrition (for 100g):

314 Calories

22.8g Fat

12.1g Carbohydrates

21.7g Protein

609mg Sodium

31.6g Fat

33.1g Carbohydrates

8g Protein

654mg Sodium

288. Salad with Roquefort Cheese

Preparation Time: 20 minutes

Cooking Time: 25 minutes

Servings: 6

Ingredients:

- 1 leaf lettuce, torn into bite-sized pieces
- 3 pears - peeled, without a core and cut into pieces
- 5 oz Roquefort cheese, crumbled
- 1/2 cup chopped green onions
- 1 avocado - peeled, seeded and diced
- 1/4 cup white sugar
- 1/2 cup pecan nuts
- 1 1/2 teaspoon white sugar
- 1/3 cup olive oil,
- 3 tablespoons red wine vinegar,
- 1 1/2 teaspoons prepared mustard,
- 1 clove of chopped garlic,
- 1/2 teaspoon ground fresh black pepper

Directions:

1. Incorporate 1/4 cup of sugar with the pecans in a frying pan over medium heat. Continue to stir gently until the sugar has melted with pecans. Carefully situate the nuts to wax paper. Set aside and break into pieces.
2. Combination for vinaigrette oil, vinegar, 1 1/2 teaspoon of sugar, mustard, chopped garlic, salt, and pepper.
3. In a large bowl, mix lettuce, pears, blue cheese, avocado, and green onions. Pour vinaigrette over salad, topped with pecans and serve.

Nutrition (for 100g):

426 Calories

Meat

289. Squash Soup with Peppers

Preparation Time: 15 minutes

Cooking Time: 20 minutes

Servings: 2

Ingredients:

- ½ lb. butternut squash, chunks
- 1 cup kale, torn
- 1 red bell pepper, chopped
- 1 cup yellow bell pepper, chopped
- 5-6 green pitted olives
- 2 stalks celery, chopped
- 4 cups water
- 1 tsp. oregano
- 1 tsp. Dijon mustard
- Pinch of salt and white pepper

Directions:

1. Boil 4 cups of water in a large saucepan. Lower the heat to medium.
2. Add the cubed squash, chopped bell peppers, kale, celery, olives, salt and spices.
3. Cover with the lid and let the soup simmer for 15 minutes. Cool and blend to a smooth paste.
4. Top with chopped parsley leaves, spring onion, seeds, or nuts. Serve hot with toasted bread, baked nachos, or crackers.

Nutrition:

Calories: 51

Protein: 1.3g

Fats: 0.3g

Carbohydrates: 9.7g

290. Grilled Steak, Mushroom and Onion Kebabs

Preparation Time: 10 minutes

Cooking Time: 10 minutes

Servings: 2

Ingredients:

- 1 lb. boneless top sirloin steak
- 8 oz. white button mushrooms
- 1 medium red onion
- 4 peeled garlic cloves
- 2 rosemary sprigs
- 2 tsps. extra-virgin olive oil
- ¼ tsp. black pepper.
- 2 tsps. red wine vinegar
- ¼ tsp. sea salt

Directions:

1. Soak 12 (10-inch) wooden skewers in water. Spray the cold grill with nonstick cooking spray and heat the grill to medium-high.
2. Cut a piece of aluminum foil into a 10-inch square. Place the garlic and rosemary sprigs in the center, drizzle with 1 tbsp. of oil and wrap tightly to form a foil packet.
3. Arrange it on the grill and seal the grill cover.
4. Cut the steak into 1-inch cubes. Thread the beef onto the wet skewers, alternating with whole mushrooms and onion wedges. Spray the kebabs thoroughly with nonstick cooking spray and sprinkle with pepper.
5. Cook the kebabs on the covered grill for 5 minutes.
6. Flip and grill for 5 more minutes while covered.
7. Unwrap foil packets with garlic and rosemary sprigs and put them into a small bowl.
8. Carefully strip the rosemary sprigs of their leaves into the bowl and pour in any accumulated juices and oil from the foil packet.
9. Mix in the remaining 1 tbsp. of oil and the vinegar and salt.
10. Mash the garlic with a fork, and mix all the ingredients in the bowl together. Pour over the finished steak kebabs and serve.

Nutrition:

Calories: 410

Protein: 36g

Fats: 14g

Carbohydrates: 12g

291. Mediterranean Lamb Chops

Preparation Time: 10 minutes

Cooking Time: 20 minutes

Servings: 2

Ingredients:

- 4 lamb shoulder chops, 8 oz. each
- 2 tbsps. Dijon mustard
- 2 tbsps. Balsamic vinegar
- 1 tbsp. garlic, chopped
- ½ cup olive oil
- 2 tbsps. shredded fresh basil
- Pepper

Directions:

1. Pat your lamb chop dry using a kitchen towel and arrange them on a shallow glass baking dish.
2. Take a bowl and whisk in Dijon mustard, balsamic vinegar, garlic, pepper, and mix them well.
3. Whisk in the oil very slowly into the marinade until the mixture is smooth.
4. Stir in the basil.
5. Pour the marinade over the lamb chops and stir to coat both sides well.
6. Cover the chops and allow them to marinate for 1-4 hours (chilled).
7. Take the chops out and leave them for 30 minutes to allow the temperature to reach the normal level.
8. Preheat your grill to medium heat and add oil to the grate.
9. Grill the lamb chops for 5-10 minutes per side until both sides are browned.
10. Once the center of the chop reads 145°F, the chops are ready, serve it and enjoy!

Nutrition:

Calories: 521

Protein: 22g

Fats: 45g

Carbohydrates: 3.5g

292. Oven Roasted Garlic Chicken Thigh

Preparation Time: 10 minutes

Cooking Time: 55 minutes

Servings: 2

Ingredients:

- 8 chicken thighs
- Salt and pepper as needed
- 1 tbsp. extra-virgin olive oil
- 6 garlic cloves, peeled and crushed
- 1 jar (10 oz.) roasted red peppers, drained and chopped
- 1½ lbs. potatoes, diced
- 2 cups cherry tomatoes, halved
- 1/3 cup capers, sliced
- 1 tsp. dried Italian seasoning
- 1 tbsp. fresh basil

Directions:

1. Season the chicken with kosher salt and black pepper.
2. Take a cast-iron skillet over medium-high heat and heat up olive oil.
3. Sear the chicken on both sides.
4. Add the remaining ingredients except for basil and stir well.
5. Remove the heat and place a cast-iron skillet in the oven.
6. Bake for 45 minutes at 400°F until the internal temperature reaches 165°F.
7. Serve it and enjoy!

Nutrition:

Calories: 500

Protein: 35g

Fats: 23g

Carbohydrates: 37g

293. Balearic Beef Brisket Bowl

Preparation Time: 0 minutes

Cooking Time: 50 minutes

Servings: 2

- **Ingredients:** ½ cup Manto Negro dry red wine (Spanish or Mallorca dry red wine)
- 1/3 cup olives, pitted and chopped
- 14.5 oz. tomatoes with juice (diced)
- 5 garlic cloves, chopped
- ½ tsp. dried rosemary
- Salt and pepper
- 2½ lbs. beef brisket
- Olive oil
- 1 tbsp. fresh parsley, finely chopped
- 1½ cups sautéed green
- beans

Directions:

1. Pour the dry wine and olives into your slow cooker and stir in the tomatoes, garlic and rosemary.
2. Sprinkle salt and pepper to taste over the beef brisket. Place the seasoned meat on top of the wine-tomato mixture. Ladle half of the mixture over the meat. Cover the slow cooker and cook for 6 hours on High heat until fork-tender.
3. Transfer the cooked brisket to a chopping board. Tent the meat with foil and let it stand for 10 minutes.
4. Drizzle with olive oil. Cut the brisket into 6-slices across its grain. Transfer the slices to a serving platter and spoon some sauce over the meat slices. Sprinkle with parsley.
5. Serve with sautéed green beans and the remaining sauce.

Nutrition:

Calories: 370

Protein: 41g

Fats: 18g

Carbohydrates: 6g

294. Chicken Marsala

Preparation Time: 10 minutes

Cooking Time: 45 minutes

Servings: 2

Ingredients:

- 2 tbsps. olive oil
- 4 skinless, boneless chicken breast cutlets
- ¾ tbsp. black pepper, divided
- ½ tsp. kosher salt, divided
- 8 oz. mushrooms, sliced
- 4 thyme sprigs
- 0.2 quarts unsalted chicken stock
- ½ quarts Marsala wine
- tbsps. olive oil
- tbsp. fresh thyme, chopped

Directions:

1. Heat oil in a pan and fry the chicken for 4-5 minutes per side. Remove the chicken from the pan and set it aside.
2. In the same pan, add thyme, mushrooms, salt and pepper; stir fry for 1-2 minutes.
3. Add Marsala wine, chicken broth and cooked chicken. Let it simmer for 10-12 minutes on low heat.
4. Add to a serving dish.
5. Enjoy.

Nutrition:

Calories: 206

Protein: 8g

Fats: 17g

Carbohydrates: 3g

295. Herb Roasted Chicken

Preparation Time: 20 minutes

Cooking Time: 45 minutes

Servings: 2

Ingredients:

- 1 tbsp. virgin olive oil
- 1 whole chicken
- 2 rosemary springs
- 3 garlic cloves (peeled)
- 1 lemon (cut in half)
- 1 tsp. sea salt
- 1 tsp. black pepper

Directions:

1. Turn your oven to 450°F.
2. Take your whole chicken and pat it dry using paper towels. Then rub in the olive oil. Remove the leaves from 1 of the springs of rosemary and scatter them over the chicken. Sprinkle the sea salt and black pepper over the top. Place the other whole sprig of rosemary into the cavity of the chicken. Then add in the garlic cloves and lemon halves.
3. Place the chicken into a roasting pan and then place it into the oven. Allow the chicken to bake for 1 hour, check that the internal temperature should be at least 165°F. If the chicken begins to brown too much, cover it with foil and return it to the oven to finish cooking.
4. When the chicken has cooked to the appropriate temperature, remove it from the oven. Let it rest for at least 20 minutes before carving.
5. Serve with a large side of roasted or steamed vegetables or your favorite salad.

Nutrition:

Calories: 309

Protein: 27.2g

Fats: 21.3g

Carbohydrates: 1.5g

296.   Grilled Harissa Chicken

Preparation Time: 20 minutes

Cooking Time: 12 minutes

Servings: 2

Ingredients:

- 1 lemon juice
- ½ sliced red onion
- 1½ tsps. coriander
- 1½ tsps. smoked paprika
- 1 tsp. cumin
- 2 tsps. cayenne
- Olive oil
- 1½ tsps. black pepper
- Kosher salt
- 8 boneless chickens.

Directions:

1. Get a large bowl. Season your chicken with kosher salt on all sides, then add the onions, garlic, lemon juice and harissa paste to the bowl.
2. Add about 3 tablespoons of olive oil to the mixture. Heat a grill to 459 heats (an indoor or outdoor grill works just fine), then oil the grates.
3. Grill each side of the chicken for about 7 minutes. Its temperature should register 165°F on a thermometer and it should be fully cooked by then.

Nutrition:

Calories: 142.5

Protein: 22.1g

Fats: 4.7g

Carbohydrates: 1.7g

297.   Turkish Turkey Mini Meatloaves

Preparation Time: 15 minutes

Cooking Time: 20 minutes

Servings: 2

Ingredients:

- 1 lb. ground turkey breast
- 1 egg
- ¼ cup whole-wheat breadcrumbs, crushed
- ¼ cup feta cheese, plus more for topping
- ¼ cup Kalamata olives halved
- ¼ cup fresh parsley, chopped
- ¼ cup red onion, minced
- ¼ cup + 2 tbsps. hummus (refer to Homemade Hummus recipe)
- 2 garlic cloves, minced
- ½ tsp. dried basil
- ¼ tsp. dried oregano
- Salt and pepper
- ½ small cucumber, peeled, seeded, and chopped
- 1 large tomato, chopped
- 3 tbsps. fresh basil, chopped
- ½-lemon juice

- 1 tsp. extra-virgin olive oil
- Salt and pepper

Directions:

1. Preheat your oven to 425 °F.
2. Line a 5"x9" baking sheet with foil and spray the surfaces with non-stick grease. Set it aside.
3. Except for the ¼ cup of hummus, combine and mix all the turkey meatloaf ingredients in a large mixing bowl. Mix well until fully combined.
4. Divide the mixture equally into 4 portions. Form the portions into loaves. Spread a tablespoon of the remaining hummus on each meatloaf. Place the loaves on the greased baking sheet.
5. Bake for 20 minutes until the loaves no longer appear pink in the center (Ensure the meatloaf cooks through by inserting a meat thermometer and the reading reaches 165 °F).
6. Combine and mix all the topping ingredients in a small mixing bowl. Mix well until fully combined.
7. To serve, spoon the topping over the cooked meatloaves.

Nutrition:

Calories: 130

Protein: 6g

Fats: 7g

Carbohydrates: 14g

298. Lemon Caper Chicken

Preparation Time: 10 minutes

Cooking Time: 15 minutes

Servings: 2

Ingredients:

- 2 tbsps. virgin olive oil
- 2 chicken breasts (boneless, skinless, cut in half, lb. to ¾ an inch thick)
- ¼ cup capers
- 2 lemons (wedges)
- 1 tsp. oregano

- 1 tsp. basil
- ½ tsp. black pepper

Directions:

1. Take a large skillet and place it on your stove and add the olive oil to it. Turn the heat to medium and allow it to warm up.
2. As the oil heats up, season your chicken breast with the oregano, basil and black pepper on each side.
3. Place your chicken breast into the hot skillet and cook on each side for 5 minutes.
4. Transfer the chicken from the skillet to your dinner plate. Top with capers and serve with a few lemon wedges.

Nutrition:

Calories: 182

Protein: 26.6g

Fats: 8.2g

Carbohydrates:3.4g

299. Buttery Garlic Chicken

Preparation Time: 5 minutes

Cooking Time: 40 minutes

Servings: 2

Ingredients:

- 2 tbsps. ghee, melted
- 2 boneless skinless chicken breasts
- 1 tbsp. dried Italian seasoning
- 4 tbsps. butter
- ¼ cup grated Parmesan cheese
- Himalayan salt and pepper

Directions:

1. Preheat the oven to 375°F. Select a baking dish that fits both chicken breasts and coat it with ghee.
2. Pat dries the chicken breasts. Season with pink Himalayan salt, pepper, and Italian seasoning. Place the chicken in the baking dish.

3. In a medium skillet over medium heat, melt the butter. Sauté the minced garlic, for about 5 minutes.
4. Remove the butter-garlic mixture from the heat and pour it over the chicken breasts.
5. Roast in the oven for 30 to 35 minutes. Sprinkle some of the Parmesan cheese on top of each chicken breast. Let the chicken rest in the baking dish for 5 minutes.
6. Divide the chicken between 2 plates; spoon the butter sauce over the chicken and serve it.

Nutrition:

Calories: 642

Protein: 57g

Fats: 45g

Carbohydrates: 11g

300. Creamy Chicken-Spinach Skillet

Preparation Time: 10 minutes

Cooking Time: 17 minutes

Servings: 2

Ingredients:

- 1 lb. boneless skinless chicken breast
- 1 medium diced onion
- 12 oz. diced roasted red peppers
- 2 ½ cup chicken stock
- 2 cups baby spinach leaves
- 2 ½ tsp. butter
- 4 minced garlic cloves
- 7 oz. cream cheese
- Salt and pepper, to taste

Directions:

1. Place a saucepan on medium-high heat for 2 minutes. Add the butter and melt it for a minute, swirling to coat the pan.
2. Add the chicken to a pan, season with pepper and salt to taste. Cook the chicken on high heat for 3 minutes per side.
3. Lower the heat to medium and stir in the onions, red peppers and garlic. Sauté for 5

minutes and deglaze the pot with a little bit of stock.
4. Whisk in the chicken stock and cream cheese. Cook and mix until thoroughly combined.
5. Stir in the spinach and adjust the seasoning to taste. Cook for 2 minutes or until the spinach is wilted.
6. Serve it and enjoy.

Nutrition:

Calories: 484

Protein: 36g

Fats: 22g

Carbohydrates: 33g

301. Slow Cooker Meatloaf

Preparation Time: 10 minutes

Cooking Time: 6 hours and 10 minutes

Servings: 2

Ingredients:

- 2 lbs. ground bison
- 1 grated zucchini
- 2 large eggs
- Olive oil cooking spray as required
- 1 zucchini, shredded
- ½ cup parsley, fresh, finely chopped
- ½ cup parmesan cheese, shredded
- 3 tbsps. Balsamic vinegar
- 4 garlic cloves, grated
- 2 tbsps. Onion minced
- 1 tbsp. Dried oregano
- ½ tsp. Ground black pepper
- ½ tsp. Kosher salt

For the topping:

- ¼ cup shredded mozzarella cheese
- ¼ cup ketchup without sugar
- ¼ cup fresh chopped parsley

Directions:

1. Stripe line the inside of a 6-quart slow cooker with aluminum foil. Spray non-stick cooking oil over it.

173

2. In a large bowl, combine ground bison or extra-lean ground sirloin, zucchini, eggs, parsley, balsamic vinegar, garlic, dried oregano, sea or kosher salt, minced dry onion and ground black pepper.
3. Situate this mixture into the slow cooker and form an oblong-shaped loaf. Cover the cooker, set on low heat and cook for 6 hours. After cooking, open the cooker and spread ketchup all over the meatloaf.
4. Now, place the cheese above the ketchup as a new layer and close the slow cooker. Let the meatloaf sit on these 2 layers for about 10 minutes or until the cheese starts to melt. Garnish it with fresh parsley and shredded Mozzarella cheese.

Nutrition:

Calories: 320

Protein: 26g

Fats: 2g

Carbohydrates: 4g

302. Mediterranean Bowl

Preparation Time: 25 minutes

Cooking Time: 30 minutes

Servings: 2

Ingredients:

- 2 chicken breasts (chopped into 4 halves)
- 2 diced onions
- 2 bottles of lemon pepper marinade
- 2 diced green bell pepper
- 4 lemon juices
- 8 cloves of crushed garlic.
- 5 tsps. olive oil
- Feta cheese
- 1 grape tomato
- 1 large-sized diced zucchini and 1 small-sized. Otherwise, use 2 medium-sized diced zucchinis.
- Salt and pepper (according to your desired taste), 4 cups of water.
- Kalamata olives (as much as you fancy)
- 1 cup of garbanzo beans

Directions:

1. Cook the chicken breasts in boiling water for 20 minutes.
2. Sauté the onion, diced bell pepper, 1 teaspoon of garlic, olive oil and ½ lemon juice and a cup of water in a medium-sized pot for 8 minutes on medium heat.
3. After 8 minutes, add your diced chicken breast into the pot and cook for 2 more minutes on medium heat (Leave the rest of the cooking to your preferred choice).
4. Serve with feta cheese (as much as you like), ½ teaspoon of lemon pepper marinade and 1 sliced tomato on top followed by a cup of cooked garbanzo beans.
5. Serve it with 1 sliced zucchini and diced olives of your choice!

Nutrition:

Calories: 541
Protein: 34g
Fats: 4g
Carbohydrates: 45g

303. Tasty Lamb Leg

Preparation Time: 10 minutes

Cooking Time: 20 minutes

Servings: 2

Ingredients:

- 2 lbs. leg of lamb, boneless and cut into chunks
- 1 tbsp. olive oil
- 1 tbsp. garlic, sliced
- 1 cup red wine
- 1 cup onion, chopped
- 2 carrots, chopped
- 1 tsp. rosemary, chopped
- 2 tsps. thyme, chopped
- 1 tsp. oregano, chopped
- ½ cup beef stock
- 2 tbsps. tomato paste
- Pepper
- Salt

Directions:

1. Add oil into the inner pot of the instant pot and set the pot on sauté mode.
2. Add the meat and sauté until browned.
3. Add the remaining ingredients and stir well.
4. Seal the pot with the lid and cook on High for 15 minutes.
5. Once done, allow to release the pressure naturally. Remove the lid.
6. Stir well and serve it.

Nutrition:

Calories:540

Protein:65.2g

Fats: 20.4g

Carbohydrates: 10.3g

304. Mediterranean Beef Skewers

Preparation Time: 5 minutes

Cooking Time: 8 minutes

Servings: 2

Ingredients:

- 2 lbs. cubed beef sirloin.
- 3 minced garlic cloves
- 1 tbsp. fresh lemon zest
- 1 tbsp. chopped parsley
- 2 tsps. chopped thyme
- 2 tsps. minced rosemary
- 2 tsps. dried oregano
- 4 tsps. olive oil
- 2 tsps. fresh lemon juice
- Sea salt and ground black pepper, to taste

Directions:

1. Add all the ingredients, except the beef, to a bowl.
2. Preheat the grill to medium-high heat.
3. Mix in the beef to marinate for 1 hour.
4. Arrange the marinated beef onto skewers, then cook on the preheated grill for 8 minutes, flipping occasionally.
5. Once cooked, leave it aside to rest for 5 minutes; then serve it.

Nutrition:

Calories: 370

Protein: 60g

Fats: 46g

Carbohydrates: 12g

305. Turkey Meatballs

Preparation Time: 10 minutes

Cooking Time: 25 minutes

Servings: 2

Ingredients:

- ¼ diced yellow onion
- 14 oz. diced artichoke hearts
- 1 lb. ground turkey
- 1 tsp. dried parsley
- 1 tsp. oil
- 4 tsps. chopped basil.
- Pepper and salt, to taste.

Directions:

1. Grease the baking sheet and preheat the oven to 350°F.
2. On medium heat, place a nonstick medium saucepan, sauté the artichoke hearts and diced onions for 5 minutes or until onions are soft.
3. Meanwhile, in a big bowl, mix the parsley, basil and ground turkey with your hands. Season to taste.
4. Once the onion mixture has cooled, add it into the bowl and mix thoroughly.
5. With an ice cream scooper, scoop ground turkey and form balls.
6. Place on a prepared cooking sheet, pop in the oven and bake until cooked around 15-20 minutes.
7. Remove it from the pan. Serve it and enjoy.

Nutrition:

Calories: 283

Protein: 12g

Fats: 12g

Carbohydrates: 30g

306. Mushroom and Beef Risotto

Preparation Time: 5 minutes

Cooking Time: 10 minutes

Servings: 2

Ingredients:

- 2 cups low-sodium beef stock
- 2 cups water
- 2 tbsps. olive oil
- ½ cup scallions, chopped
- 1 cup Arborio rice
- 1 cup roast beef, thinly stripped
- ½ cup canned cream of mushroom
- Salt and pepper as needed
- Oregano, chopped
- Parsley, chopped

Directions:

1. Take a stockpot and put it over medium heat.
2. Add water with beef stock in it.
3. Bring the mixture to a boil and remove the heat.
4. Take another heavy-bottomed saucepan and put it over medium heat.
5. Add in the scallions and stir fry them for 1 minute.
6. Add in the rice and cook it for at least 2 minutes, occasionally stirring it to ensure that it is finely coated with oil.
7. In the rice mixture, keep adding your beef stock, ½ cup at a time, making sure to stir it often.
8. Once all the stock has been added, cook the rice for another 2 minutes.
9. During the last 5 minutes of your cooking, make sure to add the beef, cream of the mushroom while stirring it nicely.
10. Transfer the whole mix to a serving dish.
11. Garnish with some chopped-up parsley and oregano. Serve it hot.

Nutrition:

Calories: 378

Protein: 23g

Fats: 12g

Carbohydrates: 41g

307. Classic Chicken Cooking with Tomatoes and Tapenade

Preparation Time: 25 minutes

Cooking Time: 25 minutes

Servings: 2

Ingredients:

- 4-5 oz. chicken breasts, boneless and skinless
- ¼ tsp. salt (divided)
- 3 tbsps. fresh basil leaves, chopped (divided)
- 1 tbsp. olive oil
- 1½ cups cherry tomatoes halved
- ¼ cup olive tapenade

Directions:

1. Arrange the chicken on a sheet of glassine or waxed paper. Sprinkle half of the salt and a third of the basil evenly over the chicken.
2. Press lightly and flip over the chicken pieces. Sprinkle the remaining salt and another third of the basil. Cover the seasoned chicken with another sheet of waxed paper.
3. Using a meat mallet or rolling pin, reduce 1 pound of the chicken to a half-inch thickness.
4. Heat the olive oil in a 12-inch skillet placed over medium-high heat. Add the pounded chicken breasts.
5. Cook for 6 minutes on each side until the chicken turns golden brown with no traces of pink in the middle. Transfer the browned chicken breasts to a platter and cover to keep them warm.
6. In the same skillet, add the olive tapenade and tomatoes. Cook for 3 minutes until the tomatoes just begin to be tender.
7. To serve, pour over the tomato-tapenade mixture over the cooked chicken breasts and top with the remaining basil.

Nutrition:

Calories: 190
Protein: 26g
Fats: 7g
Carbohydrates: 6g

308.   Grilled Grapes and Chicken Chunks

Preparation Time: 15 minutes

Cooking Time: 30 minutes

Servings: 2

Ingredients:

- 2 garlic cloves, minced
- ¼ cup extra-virgin olive oil
- 1 tbsp. rosemary, minced
- 1 tbsp. oregano, minced
- 1 tsp. lemon zest
- ½ tsp. red chili flakes, crushed
- 1 lb. chicken breast, boneless and skinless
- 1¾ cups green grapes, seedless and rinsed
- ½ tsp. salt
- 1 tbsp. lemon juice
- 2 tbsps. extra-virgin olive oil

Directions:

1. Combine and mix all the marinade ingredients in a small mixing bowl. Mix them well until fully combined. Set it aside.
2. Cut the chicken breast into ¾-inch cubes. Alternately, thread the chicken and grapes onto 12 skewers. Place the skewers in a large baking dish to hold them for marinating.
3. Pour the marinade over the skewers, coating them thoroughly. Marinate for 4 to 24 hours.
4. Remove the skewers from the marinade and allow to drip off any excess oil. Sprinkle over with salt.
5. Grill the chicken and grape skewers for 3 minutes on each side until cooked through.

6. To serve, arrange the skewers on a serving platter and drizzle with lemon juice and olive oil.

Nutrition:

Calories: 230

Protein: 1g

Fats: 20g

Carbohydrates: 14g

309.   Beef and Bulgur Meatballs

Preparation Time: 20 minutes

Cooking Time: 28 minutes

Servings: 2

Ingredients:

- ¾ cup uncooked bulgur
- 1 lb. ground beef
- ¼ cup shallots, minced
- ¼ cup fresh parsley, minced
- ½ tsp. ground allspice
- ½ tsp. ground cumin
- ½ tsp. ground cinnamon
- ¼ tsp. red pepper flakes, crushed
- Salt, as required
- 1 tbsp. olive oil

Directions:

1. In a large bowl of cold water, soak the bulgur for about 30 minutes. Drain the bulgur well and then, squeeze with your hands to remove the excess water.
2. In a food processor, add the bulgur, beef, shallot, parsley, spices, salt and pulse until a smooth mixture is formed.
3. Situate the mixture into a bowl and refrigerate it, covered, for about 30 minutes. Remove it from the refrigerator and make equal-sized balls from the beef mixture.
4. In a large nonstick skillet, heat the oil over medium-high heat and cook the meatballs in 2 batches for about 13-14 minutes, flipping frequently. Serve it warm.

Nutrition:

Calories: 228

Protein: 3.5g

Fats: 7.4g

Carbohydrates: 0.1g

310.   Italian Chicken Meatballs

Preparation Time: 20 minutes

Cooking Time: 32 minutes

Servings: 2

Ingredients:

- 3 tomatoes
- ½ cup of freshly chopped parsley
- 1 tsp. of dry oregano
- Kosher salt
- ½ tsp. of fresh thyme
- ¼ tsp. of sweet paprika
- 1 red onion
- 1 lb. of ground chicken
- ½ minced garlic cloves
- Black pepper
- 1 raw egg
- ¼ cup of freshly grated parmesan cheese
- Extra virgin olive oil

Directions:

1. Heat the oven to 375°F and get a cooking pan. Coat with extra virgin olive oil and set aside.
2. Get a large bowl and mix your tomatoes with kosher salt and thinly chopped onions.
3. Add half of your fresh thyme and sprinkle a little extra virgin olive oil on it again.
4. Transfer this to your cooking and use a spoon to spread. Add the ground chicken to the mixing bowl you recently used and add the egg, parmesan cheese and oregano.
5. Include the paprika, garlic, the other half of thyme, chopped parsley and black pepper.

6. Sprinkle a little amount of extra virgin olive oil on it and mix till the meatball mixture is combined. Form about 1½-inch chicken meatballs with the mixture and cut it all to this size.
7. Get another cooking pan and arrange these meatballs in it. Add tomatoes and onions and blend them with the meatballs. Bake in your preheated oven for about 30 minutes.
8. Your meatballs should turn golden brown, you can make them more colorful by removing them and coating them with extra virgin olive oil before you continue baking, but that is not necessary. A couple of minutes after this, your meatballs are served.
9. No surprises, your tomatoes are fast falling.

Nutrition:

Calories: 79

Protein:7.8g

Fats: 5g

Carbohydrates: 4.1g

311.   Tasty Beef and Broccoli

Preparation Time: 10 minutes

Cooking Time: 15 minutes

Servings: 2

Ingredients:

- 1½ lbs. flanks steak
- 1 tbsp. olive oil
- 1 tbsp. tamari sauce
- 1 cup beef stock
- 1 lb. broccoli, florets separated

Directions:

1. Combine the steak strips with oil and tamari, toss and set them aside for 10 minutes. Select your instant pot on sauté mode, place the beef strips and brown them for 4 minutes on each side.
2. Stir in the stock, cover the pot again and cook on High for 8 minutes. Stir in the

broccoli, cover and cook on High for 4 more minutes.

3. Divide in the plates and serve it. Enjoy!

Nutrition:

Calories: 312

Protein: 4g

Fats: 5g

Carbohydrates: 20g

312.   Grilled Chicken Breasts

Preparation Time: 10 minutes

Cooking Time: 15 minutes

Servings: 2

Ingredients:

- 4 boneless skinless chicken breasts
- 3 tsps. lemon juice
- 3 tsps. olive oil
- 3 tsps. chopped fresh parsley
- 3 minced garlic cloves
- 1 tsp. paprika.
- ½ tsp. dried oregano
- Salt and pepper, to taste.

Directions:

1. In a large Ziploc bag, mix well oregano, paprika, garlic, parsley, olive oil and lemon juice.
2. Pierce the chicken with a knife several times and sprinkle with salt and pepper.
3. Add the chicken to the bag and marinate for 20 minutes or up to 2 days in the fridge.
4. Remove the chicken from the bag and grill for 5 minutes per side in a 350°F preheated grill.
5. When cooked, transfer to a plate for 5 minutes before slicing it.
6. Serve it and enjoy with a side of rice or salad

Nutrition:

Calories: 238

Protein: 24g

Fats: 19g

Carbohydrates: 2g

313.   Charred Chicken Souvlaki Skewers

Preparation Time: 20 minutes

Cooking Time: 15 minutes

Servings: 2

Ingredients:

- ½ cup olive oil
- ½ cup fresh squeezed lemon juice
- 1 tbsp. red wine vinegar
- 1 tbsp. finely minced garlic (or garlic puree from a jar)
- 1 tbsp. dried Greek oregano
- 1 tsp. dried thyme
- 6 chicken breasts, boneless, skinless, with trimmed off tendons and **Fats:**
- Fresh cucumber and cherry tomatoes for garnish

Directions:

1. Combine and mix all the marinade ingredients in a small mixing bowl. Mix well until fully combined.
2. Slice each chicken breast crosswise into 6 1-inch strips.
3. Place the chicken strips into a large plastic container with a tight-fitting lid.
4. Pour the marinade into the plastic container, and seal with its lid. Gently shake the container and turn it over so that the marinade evenly coats all of the meat. Refrigerate the sealed plastic container to marinate for 8 hours or more.
5. Spray the grill's surfaces with non-stick grease. Preheat your charcoal or gas barbecue grill to medium-high heat.
6. Take the chicken out and let it cool to room temperature. Drain the chicken pieces and thread them onto skewers (Try to thread 6 pieces for each skewer and fold over each chicken piece so it will not spin around the skewer).

7. Grill the chicken souvlaki skewers for 15 minutes, turning once after seeing the appearance of desirable grill marks.
8. To serve, place the souvlaki on a serving plate alongside the cucumber and tomato garnish.

Nutrition:

Calories: 360

Protein: 30g

Fats: 26g

Carbohydrates: 3g

314. Slow Cooker Mediterranean Beef Roast

Preparation Time: 10 minutes

Cooking Time: 10 hours and 10 minutes

Servings: 2

Ingredients:

- 3 lbs. chuck roast, boneless
- 2 tsps. rosemary
- ½ cup tomatoes, sun-dried and chopped
- 10 cloves grated garlic
- ½ cup beef stock
- ¼ cup chopped Italian parsley, fresh
- ¼ cup chopped olives
- 1 tsp. lemon zest
- ¼ cup cheese grits

Directions:

1. In the slow cooker, put the garlic, sun-dried tomatoes and the beef roast. Add the beef stock and rosemary. Close the cooker and slow cook for 10 hours.
2. After cooking is over, remove the beef and shred the meat. Discard the fat. Add back the shredded meat to the slow cooker and simmer for 10 minutes.
3. In a small bowl combine lemon zest, parsley, and olives. Cool the mixture until you are ready to serve. Garnish it using the refrigerated mix.
4. Serve it over pasta or egg noodles. Top it with cheese grits.

Nutrition:

Calories: 314

Protein: 32g

Fats: 19g

Carbohydrates: 1g

315. Soy Sauce Beef Roast

Preparation Time: 8 minutes

Cooking Time: 35 minutes

Servings: 2

Ingredients:

- ½ tsp. beef bouillon
- 1½ tsps. rosemary
- ½ tsp. minced garlic
- 2 lbs. roast beef
- 1/3 cup soy sauce

Directions:

1. Combine the soy sauce, bouillon, rosemary and garlic together in a mixing bowl.
2. Turn on your instant pot. Place the roast and pour enough water to cover the roast; gently stir to mix well. Seal it tight.
3. Click the "Meat/Stew" cooking function; set the pressure level to "high" and set the cooking time to 35 minutes. Let the pressure build to cook the ingredients. Once done, click the "cancel" setting and click the "NPR" cooking function to release the pressure naturally.
4. Gradually open the lid and shred the meat. Mix in the shredded meat back in the potting mix and stir well. Transfer it to serving containers. Serve it warm.

Nutrition:

Calories: 423

Protein: 21g

Fats: 14g

Carbohydrates: 12g

316.   Rosemary Beef Chuck Roast

Preparation Time: 5 minutes

Cooking Time: 45 minutes

Servings: 2

Ingredients:

- 1 lb. chuck beef roast
- 1 garlic clove
- 1/8 cup balsamic vinegar
- ¼ sprig fresh rosemary
- ¼ sprig fresh thyme
- ¼ cup water
- ¼ tbsp. vegetable oil
- Salt and pepper to taste

Directions:

1. Chop slices in the beef roast and place the garlic cloves in them. Rub the roast with herbs, black pepper and salt.
2. Preheat your instant pot using the sauté setting and pour the oil. When warmed, mix in the beef roast and stir-cook until browned on all sides.
3. Add the remaining ingredients; stir gently.
4. Seal tight and cook on High for 40 minutes using a manual setting. Allow the pressure to release naturally, about 10 minutes. Uncover and put the beef roast on the serving plates, slice and serve it.

Nutrition:

Calories: 542

Protein: 55.2g

Fats: 11.2g

Carbohydrates: 8.7g

317.   Herb-Roasted Turkey Breast

Preparation Time: 15 minutes

Cooking Time: 1½ hours (plus 20 minutes to rest)

Servings: 2

Ingredients

- 2 tbsps. extra-virgin olive oil
- 4 garlic cloves, minced
- 1 lemon zest
- 1 tbsp. chopped fresh thyme leaves
- 1 tbsp. chopped fresh rosemary leaves
- 2 tbsps. chopped fresh Italian parsley leaves
- 1 tsp. ground mustard
- 1 tsp. sea salt
- ¼ tsp. freshly ground black pepper
- 1 (6 lbs.) bone-in, skin-on turkey breast
- 1 cup dry white wine

Directions:

1. Preheat the oven to 325°F. Combine the olive oil, garlic, lemon zest, thyme, rosemary, parsley, mustard, sea salt and pepper.
2. Brush the herb mixture evenly over the surface of the turkey breast and loosen the skin and rub underneath as well. Situate the turkey breast in a roasting pan on a rack, skin-side up.
3. Pour the wine into the pan. Roast for 1 to 1½ hours until the turkey reaches an internal temperature of 165°F.
4. Pull out from the oven and set it apart for 20 minutes, tented with aluminum foil to keep it warm, before carving.

Nutrition:

Calories: 392

Protein: 84g

Fats: 1g

Carbohydrates: 2g

318.   Slow Cooker Mediterranean Beef Hoagies

Preparation Time: 10 minutes

Cooking Time: 13 hours

Servings: 2

Ingredients:

- 3 lbs. beef top round roast fatless
- ½ tsp. onion powder

- ½ tsp. black pepper
- 3 cups low sodium beef broth
- 4 tsps. salad dressing mix
- 1 bay leaf
- 1 tbsp. garlic, minced
- 2 red bell peppers, thin strips cut
- 16 oz. pepperoncino
- 8 slices Sargento provolone, thin
- 2 oz. gluten-free bread
- ½ tsp. salt

For Seasoning:

- 1½ tbsp. onion powder
- 1½ tbsp. garlic powder
- 2 tbsps. dried parsley
- 1 tbsp. stevia
- ½ tsp. dried thyme
- 1 tbsp. dried oregano
- 2 tbsps. black pepper
- 1 tbsp. salt
- 6 cheese slices

Directions:

1. Dry the roast with a paper towel. Combine black pepper, onion powder and salt in a small bowl and rub the mixture over the roast.
2. Place the seasoned roast into a slow cooker.
3. Add the broth, salad dressing mix, bay leaf and garlic to the slow cooker. Combine it gently. Close and set to low cooking for 12 hours. After cooking, remove the bay leaf.
4. Take out the cooked beef and shred the beef meat. Put back the shredded beef. Add bell peppers and pepperoncino into the slow cooker.
5. Cover the cooker and low cook for 1 hour. Before serving, top each of the bread with 3 ounces of the meat mixture. Top it with a cheese slice. The liquid gravy can be used as a dip.

Nutrition:

Calories: 442

Protein: 49g

Fats: 11.5g

Carbohydrates: 37g

319.   Chicken Sausage and Peppers

Preparation Time: 10 minutes

Cooking Time: 20 minutes

Servings: 2

Ingredients:

- 2 tbsps. extra-virgin olive oil
- 6 Italian chicken sausage links
- 1 onion
- 1 red bell pepper
- 1 green bell pepper
- 3 garlic cloves, minced
- ½ cup dry white wine
- ½ tsp. sea salt
- ¼ tsp. freshly ground black pepper
- Pinch red pepper flakes

Directions:

1. Cook the olive oil on a large skillet until it shimmers. Add the sausages and cook for 5 to 7 minutes, turning occasionally, until browned and they reach an internal temperature of 165°F.
2. With tongs, remove the sausage from the pan and set it aside on a platter, tented with aluminum foil to keep warm.
3. Return the skillet to heat and mix in the onion, red bell pepper and green bell pepper. Cook and stir occasionally, until the vegetables begin to brown.
4. Put in the garlic and cook for 30 seconds, stirring constantly.
5. Stir in the wine, sea salt, pepper and red pepper flakes. Pull out and fold in any browned bits from the bottom of the pan.
6. Simmer for about 4 more minutes, stirring until the liquid reduces by half. Spoon the peppers over the sausages and serve them.

Nutrition:

Calories: 173

Protein: 22g

Fats: 1g

Carbohydrates: 6g

320. Slow Cooker Mediterranean Beef with Artichokes

Preparation Time: 3 hours and 20 minutes

Cooking Time: 7 hours and 8 minutes

Servings: 2

Ingredients:

- 2 lbs. beef for stew
- 14 oz. artichoke hearts
- 1 tbsp. grapeseed oil
- 1 diced onion
- 32 oz. beef broth
- 4 garlic cloves, grated
- 14½ oz. tinned tomatoes, diced
- 15 oz. tomato sauce
- 1 tsp. dried oregano
- ½ cup pitted, chopped olives
- 1 tsp. dried parsley
- 1 tsp. dried oregano
- ½ tsp. ground cumin
- 1 tsp. dried basil
- 1 bay leaf
- ½ tsp. salt

Directions:

1. In a large non-stick skillet, pour some oil and bring to medium-high heat. Roast the beef until it turns brown on both sides. Transfer the beef into a slow cooker.

Nutrition:

Calories: 314

Protein: 32g

Fats: 19g

Carbohydrates: 1g

321. Greek Chicken Salad

Preparation Time: 15 minutes

Cooking Time: 30 minutes

Servings: 2

Ingredients:

- ¼ cup balsamic vinegar
- 1 tsp. freshly squeezed lemon juice
- ¼ cup extra-virgin olive oil
- ¼ tsp. salt
- ¼ tsp. freshly ground black pepper
- 2 grilled boneless, skinless chicken breasts, sliced (about 1 cup)
- ½ cup thinly sliced red onion
- 10 cherry tomatoes, halved
- 8 pitted Kalamata olives, halved
- 2 cups roughly chopped romaine lettuce
- ½ cup feta cheese

Directions:

1. In a medium bowl, combine the vinegar and lemon juice and stir well. Slowly whisk in the olive oil and continue whisking vigorously until well blended. Whisk in the salt and pepper.
2. Add the chicken, onion, tomatoes and olives and stir well. Cover and refrigerate it for at least 2 hours or overnight.
3. To serve, divide the romaine between 2 salad plates and top each with half of the chicken vegetable mixture. Top with feta cheese and serve it immediately.

Nutrition:

Calories: 173

Protein: 22g

Fats: 1g

Carbohydrates: 6g

322. Chicken Piccata

Preparation Time: 10 minutes

Cooking Time: 15 minutes

Servings: 2

Ingredients:

- ½ cup whole-wheat flour
- ½ tsp. sea salt
- 1/8 tsp. freshly ground black pepper
- 1½ lbs. chicken breasts, cut into 6 pieces
- 3 tbsps. extra-virgin olive oil
- 1 cup unsalted chicken broth

- ½ cup dry white wine
- 1 lemon juice
- 1 lemon zest
- ¼ cup capers drained and rinsed
- ¼ cup chopped fresh parsley leaves

Directions:

1. In a shallow dish, whisk the flour, sea salt and pepper. Scour the chicken in the flour and tap off any excess. Cook the olive oil until it shimmers.
2. Put the chicken and cook it for about 4 minutes per side until browned. Pull out the chicken from the pan and set it aside, tented with aluminum foil to keep it warm.
3. Situate the skillet back to the heat and stir in the broth, wine, lemon juice, lemon zest and capers. Use the side of a spoon to scoop and fold in any browned bits from the pan's bottom.
4. Simmer until the liquid thickens. Take out the skillet from the heat and take the chicken back to the pan. Turn to coat. Stir in the parsley and serve.

Nutrition:

Calories: 153

Protein: 8g

Fats: 2g

Carbohydrates: 9g

323.   Grilled Calamari with Lemon Juice

Preparation Time: 10 minutes

Cooking Time: 15 minutes

Servings: 2

Ingredients:

- ¼ cup dried cranberries
- ¼ cup extra virgin olive oil
- ¼ cup olive oil
- ¼ cup sliced almonds
- 1/3 cup fresh lemon juice
- ¾ cup blueberries
- 1½ lb. or 700g cleaned calamari tube

- 1 granny smith apple, sliced thinly
- 2 tbsps. apple cider vinegar
- 6 cups fresh spinach
- Grated pepper
- Sea salt

Directions:

1. In a medium bowl, mix lemon juice, apple cider vinegar and extra virgin olive oil to make a sauce. Season with pepper and salt to taste and mix well.
2. Turn on the grill to medium fire and let the grates heat up for 1-2 minutes.
3. In a separate bowl, add the olive oil and the calamari tube. Season calamari generously with pepper and salt.
4. Place calamari onto heated grate and grill for 2-3 minutes on each side or until opaque.
5. Meanwhile, combine the almonds, cranberries, blueberries, spinach and the thinly sliced apple in a large salad bowl. Toss to mix.
6. Remove the cooked calamari from the grill and transfer to a chopping board. Cut them into ¼-inch thick rings and throw them into the salad bowl.
7. Sprinkle with already prepared sauce. Toss well to coat and serve.

Nutrition:

    Calories: 567
    Protein: 54.8g
    Fats: 24g
    Carbohydrates: 30.6g

324.   Chicken Gyros with Tzatziki

Preparation Time: 15 minutes

Cooking Time: 1 hour and 20 minutes

Servings: 2

Ingredients:

- 1 lb. ground chicken breast
- 1 onion, grated with excess water wrung out
- 2 tbsps. dried rosemary
- 1 tbsp. dried marjoram
- 6 garlic cloves, minced

- ½ tsp. sea salt
- ¼ tsp. freshly ground black pepper
- Tzatziki Sauce

Directions:

1. Preheat the oven to 350°F. Mix the chicken, onion, rosemary, marjoram, garlic, sea salt and pepper using a food processor.
2. Blend until the mixture forms a paste. Alternatively, mix these ingredients in a bowl until well combined (see preparation tip).
3. Press the mixture into a loaf pan. Bake it until it reaches 165°F internal temperature. Take out from the oven and let rest for 20 minutes before slicing.
4. Slice the gyro and spoon the Tzatziki sauce over the top.

Nutrition:

Calories: 289

Protein: 50g

Fats: 1g

Carbohydrates: 20g

325. 1-Pot Greek Chicken and Lemon Rice

Preparation Time: 15 minutes

Cooking Time: 45 minutes

Servings: 2

Ingredients:

Chicken and Marinade:

- 2 chicken thighs, skin on, bone
- ½ lemon, use the zest + 1 tbsp. lemon juice
- ½ tbsp. dried oregano
- 1 garlic clove, minced
- Salt

Rice:

- ¼ tbsp. olive oil, separated
- ½ small onion, finely diced

- ¼ cup long-grain rice, uncooked
- ½ cup chicken broth/stock
- ¼ cup water
- ½ tbsp. dried oregano
- Salt
- Black pepper
- Garnish
- Finely chopped parsley or oregano (optional)
- Fresh lemon zest (highly recommended)

Directions:

1. Combine the chicken and marinade ingredients in a Ziploc bag and set it aside for at least 20 minutes, but preferably overnight.

To Cook:

2. Preheat the oven to 180°C/350°F.
3. Remove the chicken from the marinade, but reserve the marinade.
4. Heat ½ tablespoons of olive oil in a deep, heavy-based skillet over medium-high heat.
5. Place the chicken in the skillet, skin side down, and cook until golden brown, then turn and cook the other side until golden brown.
6. Remove the chicken and set it aside.
7. Pour off the fat and wipe the pan with a scrunched-up ball of paper towel (to remove black bits), then return to the stove.
8. Heat 1 tablespoon of olive oil in the skillet over medium-high heat. Add the onion and sauté for a few minutes until translucent.
9. Then add the remaining rice ingredients and reserved marinade.
10. Let the liquid come to a simmer and let it simmer for 30 seconds. Place the chicken on top; then place a lid on the skillet.
11. Bake in the oven for 35 minutes. Then, remove the lid and bake for a further 10 minutes, or until all the liquid is absorbed and the rice is tender (so 45 minutes in total).
12. Remove it from the oven, allowing it to rest for 5 to 10 minutes before serving garnished with parsley or oregano and fresh lemon zest if desired.

Nutrition:

Calories: 173

Protein: 22g

Fats: 1g

Carbohydrates: 6g

326. Balsamic Beef Dish

Preparation Time: 15 minutes

Cooking Time: 45 minutes

Servings: 2

Ingredients:

- 3 lbs. or 1360g chuck roast
- 3 garlic cloves, sliced
- 1 tbsp. oil
- 1 tsp. flavored vinegar
- ½ tsp. pepper
- ½ tsp. rosemary
- 1 tbsp. butter
- ½ tsp. thyme
- 1 cup beef broth

Directions:

1. Slice openings in the roast and stuff them with garlic slices.
2. Using a bowl, combine pepper, vinegar and rosemary. Rub all over the roast.
3. Place your pot on the heat. Add in the oil and heat on sauté mode.
4. Add in the roast and cook until both sides brown (each side to take 5 minutes). Remove from the pot and set it aside.
5. Add in thyme, broth, butter and deglaze your pot.
6. Set back the roast and cook for 40 minutes on high heat while covered.
7. Remove the lid and serve it!

Nutrition:

Calories: 393

Protein:37g

Fats: 15g

Carbohydrates: 25g

327. Greek Chicken with Vegetables and Lemon Vinaigrette

Preparation Time: 15 minutes

Cooking Time: 50 minutes

Servings: 2

Ingredients:

For the Lemon Vinaigrette:

- 1 tsp. lemon zest
- 1 tbsp. lemon juice
- 1 tbsp. olive oil
- 1 tbsp. crumbled feta cheese
- ½ tsp. honey

For the Greek Chicken and Roasted Veggies:

- 8 oz. or 226.7g boneless chicken breast, skinless and halved
- ¼ cup light mayonnaise
- 2 cloves minced garlic
- ½ cup panko bread crumbs
- 3 tbsps. Parmesan cheese, grated
- ½ tsp. kosher salt
- ½ tsp. black pepper
- 1 tbsp. olive oil
- ½ cup dill sliced

Directions:

1. To make the vinaigrette, put a teaspoon of zest, 1 tablespoon of lemon juice, olive oil, cheese and honey in a bowl.
2. For the vegetables and chicken, preheat the oven to 470°F/243°C. Use a meat mallet for flattening the chicken into 2 pieces.
3. Using a bowl, set in the chicken. Add in 2 garlic cloves and mayonnaise. Mix the cheese, bread crumbs, pepper and salt together. Dip the chicken in this crumb mix. Spray olive oil over the chicken.
4. Roast in the oven till the chicken is done and vegetables are tender. Sprinkle dill over it and serve.

Nutrition:

Calories: 306

Protein:30g

Fats: 15g

Carbohydrates: 12g

328. Simple Grilled Salmon with Veggies

Preparation Time: 10 minutes

Cooking Time: 25 minutes

Servings: 2

Ingredients:

- 1 halved zucchini
- 2 trimmed oranges, red or yellow bell peppers, halved and seeded
- 1 red onion, wedged
- 1 tbsp. olive oil
- ½ tsp. salt and ground pepper
- 1¼ lbs. or 0.57kg salmon fillet, 4 slices
- ¼ cup sliced fresh basil
- 1 lemon, wedged

Directions:

1. Preheat the grill to medium-high. Brush the peppers, zucchini and onion with oil. Sprinkle a ¼ tsp. of salt over it. Sprinkle the salmon with salt and pepper.
2. Place the veggies and the salmon on the grill. Cook the veggies for 6 to 8 minutes on each side, till the grill marks appear. Cook the salmon till it flakes when you test it with a fork.
3. When cooled down, chop the veggies roughly and mix them in a bowl. You can remove the salmon skin to serve it with the veggies.
4. Each serving can be garnished with a tablespoon of basil and a lemon wedge.

Nutrition:

Calories: 281

Protein: 30g

Fats: 13g

Carbohydrates: 11g

329. Caprese Chicken Hasselback Style

Preparation Time: 10 minutes

Cooking Time: 30 minutes

Servings: 2

Ingredients:

- 2 (8 oz. or 226.7g each) skinless chicken breasts, boneless
- ½ tsp. salt
- ½ tsp. ground pepper
- 1 sliced tomato
- 3 oz. or 85g fresh mozzarella, halved and sliced
- ¼ cup prepared pesto
- 8 cups broccoli florets
- 2 tbsps. olive oil

Directions:

1. Set your oven to 375°F/190°C and coat a rimmed baking sheet with cooking spray.
2. Make crosswire cuts at half inches in the chicken breasts. Sprinkle ¼ tsp. of pepper and salt on them. Fill the cuts with mozzarella slices and tomato alternatively. Brush both the chicken breasts with pesto and put them on the baking sheet.
3. Mix the broccoli, oil, salt and pepper in a bowl. Put this mixture on 1 side of the baking sheet.
4. Bake till the broccoli is tender and the chicken is not pink in the center. Cut each of the breasts in half and serve it.

Nutrition:

> **Calories:** 355
> **Protein:** 38g
> **Fats:** 19g
> **Carbohydrates:** 4g

330. Bacon-Wrapped Chicken

Preparation Time: 10 minutes

Cooking Time: 50 minutes

Servings: 2

Ingredients:

- 4 slices bacon
- Salt
- Pepper
- 4 oz. or 113g Cheddar cheese, grated
- 2 chicken breasts
- Paprika to taste
- 2 tbsps. lemon or orange fresh juice

Directions:

1. Heat the oven to 350°F/176°C.
2. Place the chicken breasts into a medium bowl and season with salt, pepper, paprika and fresh juice.
3. Replace the chicken breasts with a baking pan.
4. Add cheese on top and place bacon slices over chicken breasts.
5. Place the baking pan in the oven for 45 minutes.
6. Withdraw from the oven your dish and the double-meat meal are ready to be served.

Note: If you want to get extra crispy bacon, place your cooked breasts covered with cheese and bacon on a grill or skillet and sauté for 2 minutes on each side.

Nutrition:

Calories: 206

Protein:30g

Fats: 8g

Carbohydrates: 1.6g

331. Broccoli Pesto Spaghetti

Preparation Time: 10 minutes

Cooking Time: 20 minutes

Servings: 2

Ingredients:

- 8 oz. or 226.7g spaghetti
- 1 lb. or 450g broccoli, cut into florets
- 2 tbsps. olive oil
- 4 garlic cloves, chopped
- 4 basil leaves
- 2 tbsps. blanched almonds
- 1 juiced lemon
- Salt and pepper

Directions:

1. For the pesto, combine the broccoli, oil, garlic, basil, lemon juice and almonds in a blender and pulse until well mixed and smooth.
2. Set the spaghetti in a pot, add salt and pepper. Cook until al dente for about 8 minutes. Drain it well.
3. Mix the warm spaghetti with the broccoli pesto and serve it.

Nutrition:

Calories: 284

Protein:10.4g

Fats: 10.2g

Carbohydrates: 40.2g

Bread and Pizza Recipes

332.   Avocado and Turkey Mix Panini

Preparation Time: 5 minutes

Cooking Time: 8 minutes

Servings: 2

Ingredients:

- 2 red peppers, roasted and sliced into strips
- ¼ lb. thinly sliced mesquite smoked turkey breast
- 1 cup whole fresh spinach leaves, divided
- 2 slices provolone cheese
- 1 tbsp olive oil, divided
- 2 ciabatta rolls
- ¼ cup mayonnaise
- ½ ripe avocado

Directions:

1. In a bowl, mash thoroughly together mayonnaise and avocado. Then preheat Panini press.
2. Chop the bread rolls in half and spread olive oil on the insides of the bread. Then fill it with filling, layering them as you go: provolone, turkey breast, roasted red pepper, spinach leaves and spread avocado mixture and cover with the other bread slice.
3. Place sandwich in the Panini press and grill for 5 to 8 minutes until cheese has melted and bread is crisped and ridged.

Nutrition (for 100g):

546 Calories

34.8g Fat

31.9g Carbohydrates

27.8g Protein

582mg Sodium

333.   Cucumber, Chicken and Mango Wrap

Preparation Time: 5 minutes

Cooking Time: 20 minutes

Serving: 1

Ingredients:

- ½ of a medium cucumber cut lengthwise
- ½ of ripe mango
- 1 tbsp salad dressing of choice
- 1 whole wheat tortilla wrap
- 1-inch thick slice of chicken breast around 6-inch in length
- 2 tbsp oil for frying
- 2 tbsp whole wheat flour
- 2 to 4 lettuce leaves
- Salt and pepper to taste

Directions:

1. Slice a chicken breast into 1-inch strips and just cook a total of 6-inch strips. That would be like two strips of chicken. Store remaining chicken for future use.
2. Season chicken with pepper and salt. Dredge in whole wheat flour.
3. On medium fire, place a small and nonstick fry pan and heat oil. Once oil is hot, add chicken strips and fry until golden brown around 5 minutes per side.
4. While chicken is cooking, place tortilla wraps in oven and cook for 3 to 5 minutes. Then set aside and transfer in a plate.
5. Slice cucumber lengthwise, use only ½ of it and store remaining cucumber. Peel cucumber cut into quarter and remove pith. Place the two slices of cucumber on the tortilla wrap, 1-inch away from the edge.
6. Slice mango and store the other half with seed. Peel the mango without seed, slice into strips and place on top of the cucumber on the tortilla wrap.
7. Once chicken is cooked, place chicken beside the cucumber in a line.
8. Add cucumber leaf, drizzle with salad dressing of choice.
9. Roll the tortilla wrap, serve and enjoy.

Nutrition (for 100g):

434 Calories

10g Fat

65g Carbohydrates

21g Protein

691mg Sodium

334. Fattoush –Middle East Bread

Preparation Time: 10 minutes

Cooking Time: 15 minutes

Servings: 6

Ingredients:

- 2 loaves pita bread
- 1 tbsp Extra Virgin Olive Oil
- 1/2 tsp sumac, more for later
- Salt and pepper
- 1 heart of Romaine lettuce
- 1 English cucumber
- 5 Roma tomatoes
- 5 green onions
- 5 radishes
- 2 cups chopped fresh parsley leaves
- 1 cup chopped fresh mint leaves

Dressing **Ingredients:**

- 1 1/2 lime, juice of
- 1/3 cup Extra Virgin Olive Oil
- Salt and pepper
- 1 tsp ground sumac
- 1/4 tsp ground cinnamon
- scant 1/4 tsp ground allspice

Directions:

1. For 5 minutes toast the pita bread in the toaster oven. And then break the pita bread into pieces.
2. In a large pan on medium fire, heat 3 tbsp of olive oil in for 3 minutes. Add pita bread and fry until browned, around 4 minutes while tossing around.

3. Add salt, pepper and 1/2 tsp of sumac. Set aside the pita chips from the heat and put in paper towels to drain.
4. Toss well the chopped lettuce, cucumber, tomatoes, green onions, sliced radish, mint leaves and parsley in a large salad bowl.
5. To make the lime vinaigrette, whisk together all ingredients in a small bowl.
6. Stir in the dressing onto the salad and toss well. Mix in the pita bread.
7. Serve and enjoy.

Nutrition (for 100g):

192 Calories

13.8g Fats

16.1g Carbohydrates

3.9g Protein

655mg Sodium

335. Garlic & Tomato Gluten Free Focaccia

Preparation Time: 5 minutes

Cooking Time: 20 minutes

Serving: 8

Ingredients:

- 1 egg
- ½ tsp lemon juice
- 1 tbsp honey
- 4 tbsp olive oil
- A pinch of sugar
- 1 ¼ cup warm water
- 1 tbsp active dry yeast
- 2 tsp rosemary, chopped
- 2 tsp thyme, chopped
- 2 tsp basil, chopped
- 2 cloves garlic, minced
- 1 ¼ tsp sea salt
- 2 tsp xanthan gum
- ½ cup millet flour
- 1 cup potato starch, not flour
- 1 cup sorghum flour
- Gluten free cornmeal for dusting

Directions:

1. For 5 minutes, turn on the oven and then turn it off, while keeping oven door closed.
2. Combine warm water and pinch of sugar. Add yeast and swirl gently. Leave for 7 minutes.
3. In a large mixing bowl, whisk well herbs, garlic, salt, xanthan gum, starch, and flours. Once yeast is done proofing, pour into bowl of flours. Whisk in egg, lemon juice, honey, and olive oil.
4. Mix thoroughly and place in a well-greased square pan, dusted with cornmeal. Top with fresh garlic, more herbs, and sliced tomatoes. Place in the warmed oven and let it rise for half an hour.
5. Turn on oven to 375oF and after preheating time it for 20 minutes. Focaccia is done once tops are lightly browned. Remove from oven and pan immediately and let it cool. Best served when warm.

Nutrition (for 100g):

251 Calories

9g Fat

38.4g Carbohydrates

5.4g Protein

366mg Sodium

336. Grilled Burgers with Mushrooms

Preparation Time: 15 minutes

Cooking Time: 10 minutes

Serving: 4

Ingredients:

- 2 Bibb lettuce, halved
- 4 slices red onion
- 4 slices tomato
- 4 whole wheat buns, toasted
- 2 tbsp olive oil
- ¼ tsp cayenne pepper, optional
- 1 garlic clove, minced

- 1 tbsp sugar
- ½ cup water
- 1/3 cup balsamic vinegar
- 4 large Portobello mushroom caps, around 5-inches in diameter

Directions:

1. Remove stems from mushrooms and clean with a damp cloth. Transfer into a baking dish with gill-side up.
2. In a bowl, mix thoroughly olive oil, cayenne pepper, garlic, sugar, water and vinegar. Pour over mushrooms and marinate mushrooms in the ref for at least an hour.
3. Once the one hour is nearly up, preheat grill to medium high fire and grease grill grate.
4. Grill mushrooms for five minutes per side or until tender. Baste mushrooms with marinade so it doesn't dry up.
5. To assemble, place ½ of bread bun on a plate, top with a slice of onion, mushroom, tomato and one lettuce leaf. Cover with the other top half of the bun. Repeat process with remaining ingredients, serve and enjoy.

Nutrition (for 100g):

244 Calories

9.3g Fat

32g Carbohydrates

8.1g Protein

693mg Sodium

337. Mediterranean Baba Ghanoush

Preparation Time: 10 minutes

Cooking Time: 25 minutes

Serving: 4

Ingredients:

- 1 bulb garlic
- 1 red bell pepper, halved and seeded
- 1 tbsp chopped fresh basil
- 1 tbsp olive oil

- 1 tsp black pepper
- 2 eggplants, sliced lengthwise
- 2 rounds of flatbread or pita
- Juice of 1 lemon

Directions:

1. Brush grill grate with cooking spray and preheat grill to medium high.
2. Slice tops of garlic bulb and wrap in foil. Place in the cooler portion of the grill and roast for at least 20 minutes. Place bell pepper and eggplant slices on the hottest part of grill. Grill for both sides.
3. Once bulbs are done, peel off skins of roasted garlic and place peeled garlic into food processor. Add olive oil, pepper, basil, lemon juice, grilled red bell pepper and grilled eggplant. Puree and pour into a bowl.
4. Grill bread at least 30 seconds per side to warm. Serve bread with the pureed dip and enjoy.

Nutrition (for 100g):

231.6 Calories

4.8g Fat

36.3g Carbohydrates

6.3g Protein

593mg Sodium

338. Multi Grain & Gluten Free Dinner Rolls

Preparation Time: 10 minutes

Cooking Time: 20 minutes

Serving: 8

Ingredients:

- ½ tsp apple cider vinegar
- 3 tbsp olive oil
- 2 eggs
- 1 tsp baking powder
- 1 tsp salt
- 2 tsp xanthan gum
- ½ cup tapioca starch

- ¼ cup brown teff flour
- ¼ cup flax meal
- ¼ cup amaranth flour
- ¼ cup sorghum flour
- ¾ cup brown rice flour

Directions:

1. Mix well water and honey in a small bowl and add yeast. Leave it for exactly 10 minutes.
2. Combine the following with a paddle mixer: baking powder, salt, xanthan gum, flax meal, sorghum flour, teff flour, tapioca starch, amaranth flour, and brown rice flour.
3. In a medium bowl, whisk well vinegar, olive oil, and eggs.
4. Into bowl of dry ingredients pour in vinegar and yeast mixture and mix well.
5. Grease a 12-muffin tin with cooking spray. Transfer dough evenly into 12 muffin tins and leave it for an hour to rise.
6. Then preheat oven to 375oF and bake dinner rolls until tops are golden brown, around 20 minutes.
7. Remove dinner rolls from oven and muffin tins immediately and let it cool.
8. Best served when warm.

Nutrition (for 100g):

207 Calories

8.3g Fat

27.8g Carbohydrates

4.6g Protein

844mg Sodium

339. Quinoa Pizza Muffins

Preparation Time: 15 minutes

Cooking Time: 30 minutes

Serving: 4

Ingredients:

- 1 cup uncooked quinoa
- 2 large eggs

- ½ medium onion, diced
- 1 cup diced bell pepper
- 1 cup shredded mozzarella cheese
- 1 tbsp dried basil
- 1 tbsp dried oregano
- 2 tsp garlic powder
- 1/8 tsp salt
- 1 tsp crushed red peppers
- ½ cup roasted red pepper, chopped*
- Pizza Sauce, about 1-2 cups

Directions:

1. Preheat oven to 350oF. Cook quinoa according to directions. Combine all ingredients (except sauce) into bowl. Mix all ingredients well.
2. Scoop quinoa pizza mixture into muffin tin evenly. Makes 12 muffins. Bake for 30 minutes until muffins turn golden in color and the edges are getting crispy.
3. Top with 1 or 2 tbsp pizza sauce and enjoy!

Nutrition (for 100g):

303 Calories

6.1g Fat

41.3g Carbohydrates

21g Protein

694mg Sodium

340.   Rosemary-Walnut Loaf Bread

Preparation Time: 5 minutes

Cooking Time: 45 minutes

Serving: 8

Ingredients:

- ½ cup chopped walnuts
- 4 tbsp fresh, chopped rosemary
- 1 1/3 cups lukewarm carbonated water
- 1 tbsp honey
- ½ cup extra virgin olive oil
- 1 tsp apple cider vinegar
- 3 eggs

- 5 tsp instant dry yeast granules
- 1 tsp salt
- 1 tbsp xanthan gum
- ¼ cup buttermilk powder
- 1 cup white rice flour
- 1 cup tapioca starch
- 1 cup arrowroot starch
- 1 ¼ cups all-purpose Bob's Red Mill gluten-free flour mix

Directions:

1. In a large mixing bowl, whisk well eggs. Add 1 cup warm water, honey, olive oil, and vinegar.
2. While beating continuously, incorporate the rest of the ingredients except for rosemary and walnuts.
3. Continue beating. If dough is too firm, stir a bit of warm water. Dough should be shaggy and thick.
4. Then add rosemary and walnuts continue kneading until evenly distributed.
5. Cover bowl of dough with a clean towel, place in a warm spot, and let it rise for 30 minutes.
6. Fifteen minutes into rising time, preheat oven to 400oF.
7. Generously grease with olive oil a 2-quart Dutch oven and preheat inside oven without the lid.
8. Once dough is done rising, remove pot from oven, and place dough inside. With a wet spatula, spread top of dough evenly in pot.
9. Brush tops of bread with 2 tbsp of olive oil, cover Dutch oven and bake for 35 to 45 minutes. Once bread is done, remove from oven. And gently remove bread from pot. Allow bread to cool at least ten minutes before slicing. Serve and enjoy.

Nutrition (for 100g):

424 Calories

19g Fat

56.8g Carbohydrates

7g Protein

844mg Sodium

341. Tasty Crabby Panini

Preparation Time: 5 minutes

Cooking Time: 10 minutes

Servings: 4

Ingredients:

- 1 tbsp Olive oil
- French bread split and sliced diagonally
- 1 lb. shrimp crab
- ½ cup celery
- ¼ cup green onion chopped
- 1 tsp Worcestershire sauce
- 1 tsp lemon juice
- 1 tbsp Dijon mustard
- ½ cup light mayonnaise

Directions:

1. In a medium bowl mix the following thoroughly: celery, onion, Worcestershire, lemon juice, mustard and mayonnaise. Season with pepper and salt. Then gently add in the almonds and crabs.
2. Spread olive oil on sliced sides of bread and smear with crab mixture before covering with another bread slice.
3. Grill sandwich in a Panini press until bread is crisped and ridged.

Nutrition (for 100g):

248 Calories

10.9g Fat

12g Carbohydrates

24.5g Protein

845mg Sodium

342. Perfect Pizza & Pastry

Preparation Time: 35 minutes

Cooking Time: 15 minutes

Servings: 10

Ingredients:

- For the Pizza Dough:
- 2-tsp honey
- 1/4-oz. active dry yeast
- 11/4-cups warm water (about 120 °F)
- 2-tbsp olive oil
- 1-tsp sea salt
- 3-cups whole grain flour + 1/4-cup, as needed for rolling
- For the Pizza Topping:
- 1-cup pesto sauce
- 1-cup artichoke hearts
- 1-cup wilted spinach leaves
- 1-cup sun-dried tomato
- 1/2-cup Kalamata olives
- 4-oz. feta cheese
- 4-oz. mixed cheese of equal parts low-fat mozzarella, asiago, and provolone Olive oil
- Optional Topping Add-Ons:
- Bell pepper
- Chicken breast, strips Fresh basil
- Pine nuts

Directions:

1. For the Pizza Dough:
2. Preheat your oven to 350 °F.
3. Stir the honey and yeast with the warm water in your food processor with a dough attachment. Blend the mixture until fully combined. Let the mixture to rest for 5 minutes to ensure the activity of the yeast through the appearance of bubbles on the surface.
4. Pour in the olive oil. Add the salt, and blend for half a minute. Add gradually 3 cups of flour, about half a cup at a time, blending for a couple of minutes between each addition.
5. Let your processor knead the mixture for 10 minutes until smooth and elastic, sprinkling it with flour whenever necessary to prevent the dough from sticking to the processor bowl's surfaces.
6. Take the dough from the bowl. Let it stand for 15 minutes, covered with a moist, warm towel.
7. Roll out the dough to a half-inch thickness, dusting it with flour as needed. Poke holes indiscriminately on the dough using a fork to prevent crust bubbling.

8. Place the perforated, rolled dough on a pizza stone or baking sheet. Bake for 5 minutes.
9. For the Pizza Topping:
10. Lightly brush the baked pizza shell with olive oil.
11. Pour over the pesto sauce and spread thoroughly over the pizza shell's surface, leaving out a half-inch space around its edge as the crust.
12. Top the pizza with artichoke hearts, wilted spinach leaves, sun-dried tomatoes, and olives. (Top with more add-ons, as desired.) Cover the top with the cheese.
13. Put the pizza directly to the oven rack. Bake for 10 minutes until the cheese is bubbling and melting from the center to the end. Let the pizza chill for 5 minutes before slicing.

Nutrition (for 100g):

242.8 Calories

15.1g Fats

15.7g Carbohydrates

14.1g Protein

942mg Sodium

343.   Margherita Mediterranean Model

Preparation Time: 15 minutes

Cooking Time: 15 minutes

Serving: 10

Ingredients:

1-batch pizza shell

2-tbsp olive oil

1/2-cup crushed tomatoes

3-Roma tomatoes, sliced 1/4-inch thick

1/2-cup fresh basil leaves, thinly sliced

6-oz. block mozzarella, cut into 1/4-inch slices, blot-dry with a paper towel

1/2-tsp sea salt

Directions:

Preheat your oven to 450 °F.

Lightly brush the pizza shell with olive oil. Thoroughly spread the crushed tomatoes over the pizza shell, leaving a half-inch space around its edge as the crust.

Top the pizza with the Roma tomato slices, basil leaves, and mozzarella slices. Sprinkle salt over the pizza.

Transfer the pizza directly on the oven rack. Bake until the cheese melts from the center to the crust. Set aside before slicing.

Nutrition (for 100g):

251 Calories

8g Fats

34g Carbohydrates

9g Protein

844mg Sodium

344.   Frittata Filled with Zesty Zucchini & Tomato Toppings

Preparation Time: 10 minutes

Cooking Time: 15 minutes

Serving: 4

Ingredients:

- 8-pcs eggs
- 1/4-tsp red pepper, crushed
- 1/4-tsp salt
- 1-tbsp olive oil
- 1-pc small zucchini, sliced thinly lengthwise
- 1/2-cup red or yellow cherry tomatoes, halved
- 1/3 -cup walnuts, coarsely chopped
- 2-oz. bite-sized fresh mozzarella balls (bocconcini)

Directions:

1. Preheat your broiler. Meanwhile, whisk together the eggs, crushed red pepper, and salt in a medium-sized bowl. Set aside.

2. In a 10-inch broiler-proof skillet placed over medium-high heat, heat the olive oil. Arrange the slices of zucchini in an even layer on the bottom of the skillet. Cook for 3 minutes, turning them once, halfway through.
3. Top the zucchini layer with cherry tomatoes. Fill the egg mixture over vegetables in skillet. Top with walnuts and mozzarella balls.
4. Switch to medium heat. Cook until the sides begin to set. By using a spatula, lift the frittata for the uncooked portions of the egg mixture to flow underneath.
5. Place the skillet on the broiler. Broil the frittata 4-inches from the heat for 5 minutes until the top is set. To serve, cut the frittata into wedges.

Nutrition (for 100g):

284 Calories

14g Fats

4g Carbohydrates

17g Protein

788mg Sodium

345.   Banana Sour Cream Bread

Preparation Time: 10 minutes

Cooking Time: 1 hour 10 minutes

Servings: 32

Ingredients:

- White sugar (.25 cup)
- Cinnamon (1 tsp.+ 2 tsp.)
- Butter (.75)
- White sugar (3 cups)
- Eggs (3)
- Very ripe bananas, mashed (6)
- Sour cream (16 oz. container)
- Vanilla extract (2 tsp.)
- Salt (.5 tsp.)
- Baking soda (3 tsp.)
- All-purpose flour (4.5 cups)
- Optional: Chopped walnuts (1 cup)

- Also Needed: 4 - 7 by 3-inch loaf pans

Directions:

1. Set the oven to reach 300°Fahrenheit. Grease the loaf pans.
2. Sift the sugar and one teaspoon of the cinnamon. Dust the pan with the mixture.
3. Cream the butter with the rest of the sugar. Mash the bananas with the eggs, cinnamon, vanilla, sour cream, salt, baking soda, and the flour. Toss in the nuts last.
4. Dump the mixture into the pans. Bake it for one hour. Serve

Nutrition (for 100g):

263 Calories

10.4g Fat

9g Carbohydrates

3.7g Protein

633mg Sodium

346.   Homemade Pita Bread

Preparation Time: 15 minutes

Cooking Time: 5 hours (includes rising times)

Servings: 7

Ingredients:

- Dried yeast (.25 oz.)
- Sugar (.5 tsp.)
- Bread flour /mixture of all-purpose & whole wheat (2.5 cups + more for dusting)
- Salt (.5 tsp.)
- Water (.25 cup or as needed)
- Oil as needed

Directions:

1. Dissolve the yeast and sugar in ¼ of a cup lukewarm water in a small mixing container. Wait for about 15 minutes (ready when it's frothy).
2. In another container, sift the flour and salt. Make a hole in the center and add the yeast mixture (+) one cup of water. Knead the dough.

3. Situate it onto a lightly floured surface and knead.
4. Put a drop of oil into the bottom of a large bowl and roll the dough in it to cover the surface.
5. Place a dampened tea towel over the container of dough. Wrap the bowl with a damp cloth and place it in a warm spot for at least two hours or overnight. (The dough will double its size).
6. Punch the dough down and knead the bread and divide it into small balls. Flatten the balls into thick oval discs.
7. Dust a tea towel using the flour and place the oval discs on top, leaving enough room to expand between them. Powder with flour and lay another clean cloth on top. Let it rise for another one to two hours.
8. Set the oven at 425° Fahrenheit. Situate several baking sheets in the oven to heat briefly. Lightly grease the warmed baking sheets with oil and place the oval bread discs on them.
9. Sprinkle the ovals lightly with water, and bake until they are lightly browned or for six to eight minutes.
10. Serve them while they are warm. Arrange the flatbread on a wire rack and wrap them in a clean, dry cloth to keep soft for later.

Nutrition (for 100g):

210 Calories

4g Fat

6g Carbohydrates

6g Protein

881mg Sodium

347.   Flatbread Sandwiches

Preparation Time: 10 minutes

Cooking Time: 20 minutes

Serving: 6

Ingredients Needed:

- Olive oil (1 tbsp.)

- 7-Grain pilaf (8.5 oz. pkg.)
- English seedless cucumber (1 cup)
- Seeded tomato (1 cup)
- Crumbled feta cheese (.25 cup)
- Fresh lemon juice (2 tbsp.)
- Freshly cracked black pepper (.25 tsp.)
- Plain hummus (7 oz. container)
- Whole grain white flatbread wraps (3 @ 2.8 oz. each)

Directions:

1. Cook the pilaf as directed on the package instructions and cool.
2. Chop and combine the tomato, cucumber, cheese, oil, pepper, and lemon juice. Fold in the pilaf.
3. Prepare the wraps with the hummus on one side. Spoon in the pilaf and fold.
4. Slice into a sandwich and serve.

Nutrition (for 100g):

310 Calories

9g Fat

8g Carbohydrates

10g Protein

745mg Sodium

348.   Mezze Platter with Toasted Zaatar Pita Bread

Preparation Time: 10 minutes

Cooking Time: 10 minutes

Serving: 4

Ingredients:

- Whole-wheat pita rounds (4)
- Olive oil (4 tbsp.)
- Zaatar (4 tsp.)
- Greek yogurt (1 cup)
- Black pepper & Kosher salt (to your liking)
- Hummus (1 cup)
- Marinated artichoke hearts (1 cup)
- Assorted olives (2 cups)

- Sliced roasted red peppers (1 cup)
- Cherry tomatoes (2 cups)
- Salami (4 oz.)

Directions:

1. Use the medium-high heat setting to heat a large skillet.
2. Lightly grease the pita bread with the oil on each side and add the zaatar for seasoning.
3. Prepare in batches by adding the pita into a skillet and toasting until browned. It should take about two minutes on each side. Slice each of the pitas into quarters.
4. Season the yogurt with pepper and salt.
5. To assemble, divide the potatoes and add the hummus, yogurt, artichoke hearts, olives, red peppers, tomatoes, and salami.

Nutrition (for 100g):

731 Calories

48g Fat

10g Carbohydrates

26g Protein

632mg Sodium

349. Mini Chicken Shawarma

Preparation Time: 10 minutes

Cooking Time: 1 hour 15 minutes

Serving: 8

Ingredients:

- The Chicken:
- Chicken tenders (1 lb.)
- Olive oil (.25 cup)
- Lemon - zest & juice (1)
- Cumin (1 tsp.)
- Garlic powder (2 tsp.)
- Smoked paprika (.5 tsp.)
- Coriander (.75 tsp.)
- Freshly ground black pepper (1 tsp.)
- The Sauce:
- Greek yogurt (1.25 cups)
- Lemon juice (1 tbsp.)

- Grated garlic clove (1)
- Freshly chopped dill (2 tbsp.)
- Black pepper (.125 tsp/to taste)
- Kosher salt (as desired)
- Chopped fresh parsley (.25 cup)
- Red onion (half of 1)
- Romaine lettuce (4 leaves)
- English cucumber (half of 1)
- Tomatoes (2)
- Mini pita bread (16)

Directions:

1. Toss the chicken into a zipper-type baggie. Whisk the chicken fixings and add it to the bag to marinate for up to an hour.
2. Prepare the sauce by combining the juice, garlic, and yogurt in a mixing container. Stir in the dill, parsley, pepper, and salt. Place in the fridge.
3. Heat a skillet using the medium temperature heat setting. Transfer the chicken from the marinade (let the excess drip off).
4. Cook until thoroughly cooked or about four minutes per side. Chop it into bite-sized strips.
5. Thinly slice the cucumber and onion. Shred the lettuce and chop the tomatoes. Assemble and add to the pitas - the chicken, lettuce, onion, tomato, and cucumber.

Nutrition (for 100g):

216 Calories

16g Fat

9g Carbohydrates

9g Protein

745mg Sodium

350. Eggplant Pizza

Preparation Time: 10 minutes

Cooking Time: 30 minutes

Serving: 6

Ingredients:

- Eggplants (1 large or 2 medium)
- Olive oil (.33 cup)
- Black pepper & salt (as desired)
- Marinara sauce - store-bought/homemade (1.25 cups)
- Shredded mozzarella cheese (1.5 cups)
- Cherry tomatoes (2 cups - halved)
- Torn basil leaves (.5 cup)

Directions:

1. Heat the oven to reach 400° Fahrenheit. Ready the baking sheet with a layer of parchment baking paper.
2. Slice the end/ends off of the eggplant and them it into ¾-inch slices. Arrange the slices on the prepared sheet and brush both sides with olive oil. Dust with pepper and salt to your liking.
3. Roast the eggplant until tender (10 to 12 min.).
4. Transfer the tray from the oven and add two tablespoons of sauce on top of each section. Top it off with the mozzarella and three to five tomato pieces on top.
5. Bake it until the cheese is melted. The tomatoes should begin to blister in about five to seven more minutes.
6. Take the tray from the oven. Serve and garnish basil.

Nutrition (for 100g):

257 Calories

20g Fat

11g Carbohydrates

8g Protein

789mg Sodium

351. Mediterranean Whole Wheat Pizza

Preparation Time: 10 minutes

Cooking Time: 25 minutes

Serving: 4

Ingredients:

- Whole-wheat pizza crust (1)
- Basil pesto (4 oz. jar)
- Artichoke hearts (.5 cup)
- Kalamata olives (2 tbsp.)
- Pepperoncini (2 tbsp. drained)
- Feta cheese (.25 cup)

Directions:

1. Program the oven to 450° Fahrenheit.
2. Drain and pull the artichokes to pieces. Slice/chop the pepperoncini and olives.
3. Arrange the pizza crust onto a floured work surface and cover it using pesto. Arrange the artichoke, pepperoncini slices, and olives over the pizza. Lastly, crumble and add the feta.
4. Bake for 10-12 minutes. Serve.

Nutrition (for 100g):

277 Calories

18.6g Fat

8g Carbohydrates

9.7g Protein

841mg Sodium

352. Spinach & Feta Pita Bake

Preparation Time: 5 minutes

Cooking Time: 22 minutes

Serving: 6

Ingredients:

- Sun-dried tomato pesto (6 oz. tub)
- Roma - plum tomatoes (2 chopped)
- Whole-wheat pita bread (Six 6-inch)
- Spinach (1 bunch)
- Mushrooms (4 sliced)
- Grated Parmesan cheese (2 tbsp.)
- Crumbled feta cheese (.5 cup)
- Olive oil (3 tbsp.)
- Black pepper (as desired)

Directions:

1. Set the oven at 350° Fahrenheit.
2. Brush the pesto onto one side of each pita bread and arrange them onto a baking tray (pesto-side up).
3. Rinse and chop the spinach. Top the pitas with spinach, mushrooms, tomatoes, feta cheese, pepper, Parmesan cheese, pepper, and a drizzle of oil.
4. Bake in the hot oven until the pita bread is crispy (12 min.). Slice the pitas into quarters.

Nutrition (for 100g):

350 Calories

17.1g Fat

9g Carbohydrates

11.6g Protein

712mg Sodium

353.   Watermelon Feta & Balsamic Pizza

Preparation Time: 10 minutes

Cooking Time: 15 minutes

Serving: 4

Ingredients:

- Watermelon (1-inch thick from the center)
- Crumbled feta cheese (1 oz.)
- Sliced Kalamata olives (5-6)
- Mint leaves (1 tsp.)
- Balsamic glaze (.5 tbsp.)

Directions:

1. Slice the widest section of the watermelon in half. Then, slice each half into four wedges.
2. Serve on a round pie dish like a pizza round and cover with the olives, cheese, mint leaves, and glaze.

Nutrition (for 100g):

90 Calories

3g Fat

4g Carbohydrates

2g Protein

761mg Sodium

354.   Mixed Spice Burgers

Preparation Time: 10 minutes

Cooking Time: 30 minutes

Serving: 6

Ingredients:

- Medium onion (1)
- Fresh parsley (3 tbsp.)
- Clove of garlic (1)
- Ground allspice (.75 tsp.)
- Pepper (.75 tsp.)
- Ground nutmeg (.25 tsp.)
- Cinnamon (.5 tsp.)
- Salt (.5 tsp.)
- Fresh mint (2 tbsp.)
- 90% lean ground beef (1.5 lb.)
- Optional: Cold Tzatziki sauce

Directions:

1. Finely chop/mince the parsley, mint, garlic, and onions.
2. Whisk the nutmeg, salt, cinnamon, pepper, allspice, garlic, mint, parsley, and onion.
3. Add the beef and prepare six (6) 2x4-inch oblong patties.
4. Use the medium temperature setting to grill the patties or broil them four inches from the heat for 6 minutes per side.
5. When they're done, the meat thermometer will register 160° Fahrenheit. Serve with the sauce if desired.

Nutrition (for 100g):

231 Calories

9g Fat

10g Carbohydrates

32g Protein

811mg Sodium

355. Prosciutto - Lettuce - Tomato & Avocado Sandwiches

Preparation Time: 10 minutes

Cooking Time: 10 minutes

Serving: 4

Ingredients:

- Prosciutto (2 oz./8 thin slices)
- Ripe avocado (1 cut in half)
- Romaine lettuce (4 full leaves)
- Large ripe tomato (1)
- Whole grain or whole wheat bread slices (8)
- Black pepper and kosher salt (.25 tsp.)

Directions:

1. Tear the lettuce leaves into eight pieces (total). Slice the tomato into eight rounds. Toast the bread and place it on a plate.
2. Scrape out the avocado flesh from the skin and toss it to a mixing bowl. Lightly dust it using the pepper and salt. Whisk or gently mash the avocado until it's creamy. Spread over the bread.
3. Make one sandwich. Take a slice of avocado toast; top it with a lettuce leaf, a prosciutto slice, and a tomato slice. Top with another slice of lettuce tomato and continue.
4. Repeat the process until all ingredients are depleted.

Nutrition (for 100g):

240 Calories

9g Fat

8g Carbohydrates

12g Protein

811mg Sodium

356. Spinach Pie

Preparation Time: 10 minutes

Cooking Time: 60 minutes

Serving: 6

Ingredients:

- Melted butter (.5 cup)
- Frozen spinach (10 oz. pkg.)
- Fresh parsley (.5 cup)
- Green onions (.5 cup)
- Fresh dill (.5 cup)
- Crumbled feta cheese (.5 cup)
- Cream cheese (4 oz.)
- Cottage cheese (4 oz.)
- Parmesan (2 tbsp. - grated)
- Large eggs (2)
- Pepper and salt (as desired)
- Phyllo dough (40 sheets)

Directions:

1. Heat the oven setting at 350° Fahrenheit.
2. Mince/chop the onions, dill, and parsley. Thaw the spinach and sheets of dough. Dab the spinach dry by squeezing.
3. Combine the spinach, scallions, eggs, cheeses, parsley, dill, pepper, and salt in a blender until it's creamy.
4. Prepare the small phyllo triangles by filling them with one teaspoon of the spinach mixture.
5. Lightly brush the outside of the triangles with butter and arrange them with the seam-side facing downwards on an ungreased baking tray.
6. Place them in the heated oven to bake until golden brown and puffed (20-25 min.). Serve piping hot.

Nutrition (for 100g):

555 Calories

21.3g Fat

15g Carbohydrates

18.1g Protein

681mg Sodium

357. Feta Chicken Burgers

Preparation Time: 10 minutes

Cooking Time: 30 minutes

Serving: 6

Ingredients:

- ¼ cup Reduced-fat mayonnaise
- ¼ cup Finely chopped cucumber
- ¼ tsp Black pepper
- 1 tsp Garlic powder
- ½ cup Chopped roasted sweet red pepper
- ½ tsp Greek seasoning
  - lb. Lean ground chicken
- 1 cup Crumbled feta cheese
- 6 Whole wheat burger buns

Directions:

2. Preheat the broiler to the oven ahead of time. Mix the mayo and cucumber. Set aside.
3. Combine each of the seasonings and red pepper for the burgers. Mix the chicken and the cheese well. Form the mixture into 6 ½-inch thick patties.
4. Cook the burgers in a broiler and place approximately four inches from the heat source. Cook until the thermometer reaches 165° Fahrenheit.
5. Serve with buns and cucumber sauce. Garnish with tomato and lettuce if desired and serve.

Nutrition (for 100g):

356 Calories

14g Fat

10g Carbohydrates

31g Protein

691mg Sodium

358.   Roast Pork for Tacos

Preparation Time: 10 minutes

Cooking Time: 85 minutes

Serving: 6

Ingredients:

- Pork shoulder roast (4 lb.)
- Diced green chilies (2 - 4 oz. cans)
- Chili powder (.25 cup)
- Dried oregano (1 tsp.)
- Taco seasoning (1 tsp.)
- Garlic (2 tsp.)
- Salt (1.5 tsp. or as desired)

Directions:

1. Set the oven to reach 300° Fahrenheit.
2. Situate the roast on top of a large sheet of aluminum foil.
3. Drain the chilis. Mince the garlic.
4. Mix the green chilis, taco seasoning, chili powder, oregano, and garlic. Rub the mixture over the roast and cover using a layer of foil.
5. Place the wrapped pork on top of a roasting rack on a cookie sheet to catch any leaks.
6. Roast it for 3.5 to 4 hours in the hot oven until it's falling apart. Cook until the center reaches at least 145° Fahrenheit when tested with a meat thermometer (internal temperature).
7. Transfer the roast to a chopping block to shred into small pieces using two forks. Season it as desired.

Nutrition (for 100g):

290 Calories

17.6g Fat

12g Carbohydrates

25.3g Protein

359.   Italian Apple - Olive Oil Cake

Preparation Time: 10 minutes

Cooking Time: 1 hour 10 minutes

Serving: 12

Ingredients:

- Gala apples (2 large)
- Orange juice - for soaking apples
- All-purpose flour (3 cups)
- Ground cinnamon (.5 tsp.)
- Nutmeg (.5 tsp.)
- Baking powder (1 tsp.)
- Baking soda (1 tsp.)
- Sugar (1 cup)

- Olive oil (1 cup)
- Large eggs (2)
- Gold raisins (.66 cup)
- Confectioner's sugar - for dusting
- Also Needed: 9-inch baking pan

Directions:

1. Peel and finely chop the apples. Drizzle the apples with just enough orange juice to prevent browning.
2. Soak the raisins in warm water for 15 minutes and drain well.
3. Sift the baking soda, flour, baking powder, cinnamon, and nutmeg. Set it to the side for now.
4. Pour the olive oil and sugar into the bowl of a stand mixer. Mix on the low setting for 2 minutes or until well combined.
5. Blend it while running, break in the eggs one at a time and continue mixing for 2 minutes. The mixture should increase in volume; it should be thick - not runny.
6. Combine all of the ingredients well. Build hole in the center of the flour mixture and add in the olive and sugar mixture.
7. Remove the apples of any excess of juice and drain the raisins that have been soaking. Add them together with the batter, mixing well.
8. Prepare the baking pan with parchment paper. Place the batter onto the pan and level it with the back of a wooden spoon.
9. Bake it for 45 minutes at a 350° Fahrenheit.
10. When ready, remove the cake from the parchment paper and place it into a serving dish. Dust with the confectioner's sugar. Heat dark honey to garnish the top.

Nutrition (for 100g):

294 Calories

11g Fat

9g Carbohydrates

5.3g Protein

691mg Sodium

Small Plates and Snacks

360. Eggplant Caviar

Preparation Time: 10 minutes

Cooking Time: 10 minutes

Servings: 4

Ingredients:

- 2 (1-pound) eggplants
- 2 garlic cloves, mashed
- ½ cup finely chopped fresh parsley
- ½ cup finely diced red bell pepper
- ¼ cup freshly squeezed lemon juice
- 2 tablespoons tahini
- ⅛ teaspoon salt, plus more as needed

Directions:

1. Preheat the chic.
2. Pierce the eggplants with a fork to prevent them from bursting in the oven, and place them on a rimmed baking sheet. Broil for about 3 minutes until the skin is charred on one side. Flip the eggplants and broil the other side for about 3 minutes more until charred. Remove and let cool.
3. Carefully remove the skin from the eggplants and scoop the pulp into a bowl. Using a fork or wooden pestle, mash the pulp into a smooth purée.
4. Add the garlic, parsley, red bell pepper, lemon juice, tahini, and salt. Stir until well combined. Taste and then season it with more salt, as needed.
5. Refrigerate for at least 1 hour before serving. Leftover "caviar" can be kept refrigerated in an airtight container for up to 5 days, or frozen for up to 1 month. Thaw in the refrigerator overnight before using.

Nutrition:

Calories 115

Fat 5 G

Fiber 9 G

Carbs 17 G

Protein 4 G

361. Walnut and Red Pepper Spread

Preparation Time: 20 minutes

Cooking Time: 0 minutes

Servings: 6

Ingredients:

- 3 slices whole-wheat bread
- 1 red bell pepper
- ½ onion, chopped
- 1 cup walnuts
- 3 tablespoons Harissa, or store-bought
- 2 tablespoons pomegranate molasses, or cranberry juice
- ½ teaspoon ground coriander
- ½ teaspoon ground cumin
- ¼ cup olive oil

Directions:

1. In a food processor, combine the bread, red bell pepper, onion, and walnuts.
2. Process for a few seconds until combined but coarse. Do not overprocess. You want to retain some texture of the walnuts in this spread.
3. Add the harissa, molasses, coriander, cumin, and olive oil. Process it for a few seconds until the mixture resembles an almost smooth paste.
4. Refrigerate any leftovers in an airtight container for up to 1 week, or freeze for 2 to 3 months.

Nutrition:

Calories 300

Fat 24 G

Fiber 3 G

Carbs 19 G

Protein 6 G

362. Green Olive Tapenade

Preparation Time: 20 minutes

Cooking Time: 0 minutes

Servings: 6

Ingredients:

- 2 cups pitted green olives
- 1 cup coarsely chopped walnuts
- 1 onion, chopped
- ½ cup chopped fresh parsley
- ¼ cup freshly squeezed lemon juice
- ¼ cup olive oil
- 1 teaspoon dried oregano

Directions:

1. In a food processor, combine the olives, walnuts, onion, and parsley. Pulse about 5 times until the mixture is coarsely chopped.
2. Add the lemon juice, olive oil, and oregano. Process for a few seconds more. The spread should be finely chopped but not puréed.

Nutrition:

Calories 259

Fat 26 G

Fiber 3 G

Carbs 8 G

Protein 4 G

363.   Skordalia

Preparation Time: 30 minutes

Cooking Time: 0 minutes

Servings: 6

Ingredients:

- 1 cup water
- 5 large slices Italian bread, crusts removed
- 8 garlic cloves, peeled
- ⅛ teaspoon salt, plus more as needed
- 4 potatoes, peeled and boiled
- ½ cup apple cider vinegar, plus more as needed
- ½ cup olive oil

Directions:

1. Pour the water onto a rimmed baking sheet and put the bread slices into the water. Soak the bread for 5 minutes. Remove the bread and then squeeze out the excess water. Set aside.
2. In a medium bowl, using a fork or wooden pestle, mash the garlic and salt into a smooth paste. Add the boiled potatoes and soaked bread and gently mash and mix to combine.
3. Add the vinegar and olive oil and continue to mix until you have no lumps. Slowly mix in more vinegar if the skordalia is too thick to spread. Taste and then season it with more salt, as needed.
4. Cover and refrigerate until serving. Spoon any leftovers into an airtight container and freeze for up to 1 month.

Nutrition:

Calories 320

Fat 18 G

Fiber 4 G

Carbs 36 G

Protein 5 G

364.   Mint Labneh

Preparation Time: 10 minutes

Cooking Time: None

Servings: 6

Ingredients:

- 32 ounces Plain Yogurt, or store-bought
- ½ teaspoon salt
- ¼ cup olive oil
- ¼ cup finely chopped fresh mint

Directions:

1. Stir together the yogurt and salt.
2. Put a colander with some layers of cheesecloth. Put some of the yogurt mixture into the lined colander. Place the colander over a sink or a bowl and let the mixture sit for 2 hours just until most of the water is drained.

3. Spoon the labneh into a small bowl and stir in the olive oil and mint until well combined. The labneh can be refrigerated in an airtight container for 1 to 2 weeks.

Nutrition:

Calories 173

Fat 14 G

Fiber 0 G

Carbs 8 G

Protein 5 G

365. Sweet and Sour Beet Dip

Preparation Time: 10 minutes

Cooking Time: 50 minutes

Servings: 6

Ingredients:

- 1-pound beets, trimmed
- ½ cup tahini
- ½ cup freshly squeezed lemon juice
- 4 garlic cloves, mashed
- Grated zest of 1 lemon
- 1 teaspoon ground cumin
- ¼ teaspoon cayenne pepper
- Salt
- Freshly ground black pepper

Directions:

1. Mix the beets with enough water and then cover. Place the pan on high heat and boil the beets for about 50 minutes or until tender.
2. Drain the beets, let them cool, and peel them. The skins should slide off easily.
3. Transfer the beets in a food processor and purée for about 5 minutes until smooth. Transfer the puréed beets to a medium bowl.
4. Stir in the tahini, lemon juice, garlic, lemon zest, cumin, and cayenne until well mixed. Taste and then season it with some salt and black pepper, as needed.

Nutrition:

Calories 162

Fat 11 G

Fiber 4 G

Carbs 13 G

Protein 5 G

366. Marinated Olives

Preparation Time: 10 minutes

Cooking Time: None

Servings: 4

Ingredients:

- ¼ cup olive oil
- ¼ cup red wine vinegar
- Grated zest of 1 lemon
- 1 teaspoon chopped fresh rosemary
- 2 cups jarred olives, drained

Directions:

1. Whisk the olive oil, vinegar, lemon zest, and rosemary until blended.
2. Add the olives and gently stir to coat. Put well and let it marinate for at least 3 hours before serving.

Nutrition:

Calories 209

Fat 21 G

Fiber 3 G

Carbs 7 G

Protein 1 G

367. Marinated Zucchini

Preparation Time: 15 minutes

Cooking Time: 5 minutes

Servings: 6

Ingredients:

- ¼ cup balsamic vinegar
- 2 tablespoons stone-ground mustard
- 1 garlic clove, minced

- 2 teaspoons chopped fresh thyme
- ¼ cup olive oil
- ⅛ teaspoon salt
- ⅛ teaspoon freshly ground black pepper
- 3 large zucchini, cut diagonally into ½-inch-thick slices

Directions:

1. Whisk the vinegar, mustard, garlic, and thyme to combine. Whisk in the olive oil until blended. Season iwith the salt and pepper and whisk again to combine.
2. Place the zucchini in a large bowl and drizzle ¼ cup of marinade over them. Toss well to coat.
3. Heat a grill pan or sauté pan over medium heat.
4. Place the zucchini slices in the pan. Cook it for about 5 minutes, while turning occasionally, until the zucchini is tender and lightly charred.
5. Transfer the cooked zucchini back to the bowl and drizzle it with the remaining marinade. Toss to coat. Cover the bowl and refrigerate the zucchini to marinate for 30 minutes or until chilled.
6. Arrange the marinated slices on a serving platter and drizzle with the marinade from the bowl to serve.

Nutrition:

Calories 105

Fat 9 G

Fiber 2 G

Carbs 6 G

Protein 2 G

368.   Pickled Turnips

Preparation Time: 15 minutes

Cooking Time: None

Servings: 12

Ingredients:

- 4 cups water
- ¼ cup salt
- 1 cup white distilled vinegar
- 1 small beet, peeled and quartered
- 1 garlic clove, peeled
- 2 pounds turnips, peeled, halved, and cut into ¼-inch half-moons

Directions:

1. In a medium bowl, whisk the water and salt until the salt dissolves. Whisk in the vinegar.
2. Place the beet and garlic in a clean 2-quart glass jar with a tight-sealing lid. Layer the turnips on top.
3. Pour the vinegar mixture over the turnips to cover them. Seal the lid tightly and let the jar sit at room temperature for 1 week.

Nutrition:

Calories 26

Fat 0 G

Fiber 1 G

Carbs 6 G

Protein 1 G

369.   Braised Sweet Peppers

Preparation Time: 10 minutes

Cooking Time: 40 minutes

Servings: 4

Ingredients:

- ¼ cup olive oil
- 1 red onion, thinly sliced
- 3 red bell peppers
- 3 green bell peppers
- 2 garlic cloves, chopped
- ¼ teaspoon cayenne pepper
- ⅛ teaspoon salt
- ⅛ teaspoon freshly ground black pepper
- ¼ cup vegetable broth
- 1 tablespoon chopped fresh thyme

Directions:

1. Heat the olive oil.
2. Add the red onion and cook it for about 5 minutes.

3. Add the red and green bell peppers, garlic, cayenne, salt, and black pepper.
4. Pour in the vegetable broth and then bring the mixture to a boil. Cover the pan and then reduce the heat. Cook for 35 minutes, stirring occasionally, until the vegetables are soft but still firm.
5. Sprinkle the peppers with the thyme and serve.

Nutrition:

Calories 184

Fat 15 G

Fiber 4 G

Carbs 15 G

Protein 3 G

370.   Caramelized Pearl Onions

Preparation Time: 5 minutes

Cooking Time: 15 minutes

Servings: 4

Ingredients:

- ¼ cup olive oil
- 1-pound frozen pearl onions, thawed
- 3 tablespoons sugar
- ½ cup balsamic vinegar
- 1 tablespoon chopped fresh rosemary
- ⅛ teaspoon salt
- ⅛ teaspoon red pepper flakes

Directions:

1. In a sauté pan on medium heat, heat the olive oil.
2. Add the onions and then cook it for about 5 minutes until they begin to brown.
3. Add the sugar and cook for about 5 minutes more until the sugar is caramelized, gently
4. Add the vinegar and rosemary. Cook it for about 2minutes while stirring it occasionally, until a syrup forms.
5. Stir in the salt and red pepper flakes. Remove it from heat and then let it cool before serving.

Nutrition:

Calories 203

Fat 14 G

Fiber 1 G

Carbs 18 G

Protein 13 G

371.   Patatas Bravas

Preparation Time: 10 minutes

Cooking Time: 20 minutes

Servings: 4

Ingredients:

- 2 cups olive oil, divided
- 1 tablespoon cayenne pepper, plus more as needed
- 2 tablespoons sweet paprika, plus more as needed
- 1 tablespoon all-purpose flour
- 1 cup vegetable broth
- ⅛ teaspoon salt, plus more as needed
- 4 russet or Yukon Gold potatoes, peeled, cut into 1-inch cubes, and patted dry

Directions:

1. In a small saucepan over medium heat, heat ¼ cup of olive oil for about 2 minutes until warm. Remove it from the heat and then whisk in the cayenne, paprika, and flour until you have a paste.
2. Add the vegetable broth and salt. Return the saucepan to medium-low heat and then cook the mixture for about 5 minutes, stirring constantly, until it thickens into a sauce. Taste and adjust the seasoning. Remove from the heat and set the sauce aside.
3. In a large pan on medium heat, heat the remaining 1¾ cups of olive oil.
4. Gently add the potatoes and fry for about 10 minutes, stirring occasionally, until crispy and golden. Transfer the potatoes to a paper towel to drain. Transfer the potatoes to a serving platter and drizzle with the sauce.

Nutrition:

Calories 394

Fat 27 G

Fiber 7 G

Carbs 38 G

Protein 6 G

372. Dalmatian Tuna Toast

Preparation Time: 5 minutes

Cooking Time: 0 minutes

Servings: 1-2

Ingredients:

- 2 lightly toasted slices of bread
- 2 tbsp of minced tuna (you can use a fish pate instead)
- 1 tbsp of roasted chickpea

Directions:

1. Simply combine the ingredients and make this sandwich. A great tip is to spread some olive oil and crushed garlic over the bread before toasting it. This will give you a true Mediterranean flavor.

Nutrition:

Calories 40

Fat 1g

Carbs 0g

Protein 2g

373. Fish Kofte

Preparation Time: 10 minutes

Cooking Time: 25 minutes

Servings: 4

Ingredients:

- 1 lb. potato, sliced
- 7 oz fresh salmon fillet
- 1 cup of skim milk
- 1 egg

- 1 tsp of sea salt
- 1 tbsp of butter
- 1 cup of all-purpose flour
- ½ cup of breadcrumbs
- ½ cup of parsley, finely chopped
- Vegetable oil

Directions:

2. Place the potato in a deep pot. Add some enough water to cover and bring it to boil. Cook until soft. Remove from the heat and transfer to a bowl. Add one teaspoon of salt, milk, and butter. Mash until a smooth puree. Set aside.
3. Finely chop the salmon fillet and combine with potato puree. Add flour, eggs, and parsley. Mix until well combined. Using your hands, shape 1-inch thick patties and coat in breadcrumbs.
4. Preheat some oil over a medium-high heat. Fry each patty for about 5-6 minutes.

Nutrition:

Calories 487

Fat 21g

Carbs 52g

Protein 41g

374. Salty Cheese Fritters

Preparation Time: 5 minutes

Cooking Time: 15 minutes

Servings: 2-3

Ingredients:

- 1 egg
- 1 cup of yogurt
- 1 tbsp of oil
- 1 tsp of salt
- 2 tsp of baking powder
- 15 oz all-purpose flour
- Oil for frying
- Creamy Cheese
- ½ cup of gorgonzola cheese (or any blue cheese you have on hand)

- 1 cup of sour cream
- ¼ cup of grated cheddar
- 1 tbsp of finely chopped parsley
- ½ tsp of cayenne pepper

Directions:

1. Add the ingredients and mix it well with an electric mixer until you get a smooth dough.
2. Roll the dough to about one inch.
3. Cut it into 2.5x2.5inch pieces.
4. Preheat some of the oil on a medium temperature.
5. Fry the doughnuts for some several minutes on each side.
6. Served with sour cream, kefir cream, and cheese.

Nutrition:

Calories 311

Fat 29g

Carbs 51g

Protein 2g

375. Smoked Salmon Toast

Preparation Time: 5 minutes

Cooking Time: None

Servings: 2

Ingredients:

- 4 slices of toast bread (you can use any bread you have)
- 2 oz smoked salmon, thinly sliced
- 2 tbsp of olive oil
- 1 tbsp of finely chopped parsley
- 1 garlic clove, crushed
- 4 toast-sized lettuce leaves

Directions:

1. Combine the olive oil with crushed garlic and parsley. Spread this mixture over bread and lightly toast.
2. Arrange lettuce leaves and smoked salmon slices on top. Serve as breakfast.

Nutrition (Per Serving):

Calories 117

Fat 4.3g

Carbs 0g

Protein 18.2g

376. Chickpea Salad Pitas

Preparation Time: 15 minutes

Cooking Time: None

Servings: 4

Ingredients:

- o   oz chickpeas, cooked
- ½ medium-sized cucumber, sliced
- ½ small onion, finely chopped
- ½ medium-sized red bell pepper, finely chopped
- ½ cup of feta cheese, sliced
- 1 tsp of chili pepper
- ½ tsp of salt
- ½ tsp of black pepper, ground
- 2 pita breads
- HUMMUS
- 14 oz cooked chickpeas
- 2-3 tbsp lemon juice
- 2 tbsp olive oil
- 2 cloves garlic, crushed
- 1 tbsp of parsley, finely chopped
- 3 tbsp tahini

Directions:

1. Combine all ingredients in a bowl. Stir it well and then set aside for ten minutes. Cut the pitas in half and stuff with the mixture.
2. If you like, you can serve with lettuce or cherry tomatoes.

Nutrition:

Calories 180

Fat 7.2g

Carbs 31g

Protein 7g

377.   Creamy Cheese Wraps

Preparation Time: 3 minutes

Cooking Time: None

Servings: 1

Ingredients:

- 1 whole grain tortilla
- 1 medium-sized tomato
- ½ red bell pepper, finely chopped
- 1 garlic clove, crushed
- 1 tsp of dry oregano
- 2 tbsp of grated goat's cheese (can be replaced with some other cheese)
- 1 tsp of extra virgin olive oil
- ½ tsp of salt
- 2 tbsp of finely chopped parsley

Directions:

1. Spread some olive oil over tortilla and warm it up in a microwave for one minute.
2. Spread other ingredients over tortilla and wrap. Enjoy!

Nutrition:

Calories 125

Fat 6g

Carbs 29g

Protein 9.5g

378.   Tuna Durum Doner

Preparation Time: 3 minutes

Cooking Time: 1 minute

Servings: 4

Ingredients:

- 4 lettuce leaves
- 4 tbsp of sweet corn
- 2 tbsp of red beans
- 1 small tomato, finely chopped
- 2 tbsp of canned tuna, oil free
- 0.7 oz grated Gouda cheese
- ½ tsp of sea salt
- 4 corn tortillas

Directions:

1. Combine the tuna with sweet corn, red beans, grated Gouda, and finely chopped tomato.
2. Heat up tortillas in a microwave for about a minute. Spread some of the mixture on each tortilla, add lettuce and wrap. Secure with toothpicks.

Nutrition:

Calories 169

Fat 2g

Carbs 13g

Protein 9g

379.   Moroccan Breakfast Salad

Preparation Time: 15 minutes

Cooking Time: None

Servings: 2

Ingredients:

- ½ pear, sliced
- 1 kiwi, peeled and sliced
- Few cherry tomatoes, halved
- ½ cup of wild berries
- ½ cup of nut mix
- ½ green bell pepper, sliced
- DRESSING
- 2 tbsp of honey
- 1 tsp of saffron, ground
- ¼ cup of fresh lime juice
- 1 tsp of mustard

Directions:

1. Whisk fresh lime juice, saffron, mustard, and honey with a fork.
2. In a large bowl, combine the vegetables and add the dressing. Toss well to combine.

Nutrition:

Calories 36

Fat 3.5g

Carbs 7.6g

Protein 2.3g

380. Panzanella To Go

Preparation Time: 3 minutes

Cooking Time: None

Servings: 1

Ingredients:

- 2 slices of any bread
- 1 cup of finely chopped lettuce
- 1 small tomato, chopped
- 1 small onion, sliced
- ½ cucumber, sliced
- 1 tbsp of olive oil
- 1 tsp of apple cider vinegar
- ½ tsp of oregano

Directions:

1. Combine the ingredients in a bowl. Season with olive oil, apple cider, and oregano. Serve.

Nutrition:

Calories 212

Fat 11g

Carbs 35g

Protein 2g

381. Cranberries Spring Salad

Preparation Time: 15 minutes

Cooking Time: None

Servings: 2

Ingredients:

- ½ cup of cooked lentils
- ½ cup of finely chopped arugula
- ½ cucumber, sliced
- ½ orange, peeled and sectioned
- ½ carrot, sliced
- ½ green bell pepper, sliced
- ¼ cup of fresh cranberries
- BALSAMIC VINAGRETTE
- ¼ cup of olive oil
- ½ tsp of ground red pepper
- ¼ tsp of salt
- 1 tsp of balsamic vinegar

Directions:

1. Combine the vegetables in a large bowl. Add lentils and mix well. Set aside.
2. In a smaller bowl, shake together the balsamic vinegar, olive oil, salt, and red pepper. Put the vinaigrette over the vegetables and mix well. Top with orange and cranberries.
3. Serve cold.

Nutrition:

Calories 194

Fat 26g

Carbs 41g

Protein 32g

382. Cold Green Bean Salad

Preparation Time: 5 minutes

Cooking Time: 15 minutes

Servings: 2

Ingredients:

- 1 lb. green beans, trimmed
- ¼ cup of extra virgin olive oil
- 1 tbsp of Dijon mustard
- 2 garlic cloves, crushed
- 1 tbsp of lime juice

Directions:

1. Boil some water and then add one teaspoon of salt and green beans. Cook until tender. This should take about 10-15 minutes. Rinse and drain.
2. Meanwhile, combine the crushed garlic with extra virgin olive oil, Dijon, and lime juice. Drizzle over beans and serve.

Nutrition:

Calories 110

Fat 11g

Carbs 19g

Protein 4.2g

383. Greek Goat's Cheese Salad

Preparation Time: 10 minutes

Cooking Time: 12 minutes

Servings: 5

Ingredients:

- 1 cup of fresh goat's cheese
- 1 whole egg, boiled
- ½ cup of red cabbage, shredded
- Few lettuce leaves
- 1 small tomato, chopped
- 1 small onion, peeled and sliced
- ½ cucumber, peeled and sliced
- ½ red bell pepper, sliced
- Few olives
- 1 hot pepper
- ¼ cup of olive oil
- 1 tsp of mustard
- 1 tbsp of finely chopped parsley
- 1 garlic clove, crushed
- Sea salt to taste
- Black pepper to taste

Directions:

1. Combine the olive oil with mustard, finely chopped parsley, and one garlic clove. Season with some salt and pepper and mix well.
2. Place the vegetables on a serving plate. Drizzle with the olive oil dressing and serve immediately.

Nutrition:

Calories 84

Fat 7g

Carbs 9g

Protein 5g

384. Italian Seafood Salad

Preparation Time: 15 minutes

Cooking Time: 20 minutes

Servings: 2

Ingredients:

- Fresh lettuce leaves, rinsed
- 1 small cucumber, sliced
- ½ red bell pepper, sliced
- 1 cup of frozen seafood mix
- 1 onion, peeled and finely chopped
- 3 garlic cloves, crushed
- ¼ cup of fresh orange juice
- 5 tbsp of extra virgin olive oil
- Salt to taste

Directions:

1. Heat up 3 tbsp of extra virgin olive oil over medium-high temperature. Add chopped onion and crushed garlic. Stir fry for about 5 minutes. Reduce the heat to minimum and then add 1 cup of frozen seafood mix. Cover and cook for about 15 minutes, until soft. Put it away from the heat and then let it to cool for a while.
2. Meanwhile, combine the vegetables in a bowl. Add the remaining 2 table spoon of olive oil, fresh orange juice and little salt. Toss well to combine.
3. Top with seafood mix and serve immediately.

Nutrition:

Calories 286

Fat 26g

Carbs 28g

Protein 34.5g

385. Summer Squash Ribbons with Lemon and Ricotta

Preparation Time: 20 minutes

Cooking Time: None

Servings: 4

Ingredients:

- 2 medium zucchini or yellow squash
- ½ cup ricotta cheese
- 2 tablespoons fresh mint, chopped, plus additional mint leaves for garnish
- 2 tablespoons fresh parsley, chopped
- Zest of ½ lemon
- 2 teaspoons lemon juice
- ½ teaspoon kosher salt
- ¼ teaspoon freshly ground black pepper
- 1 tablespoon extra-virgin olive oil

Directions:

1. Using a vegetable peeler, make ribbons by peeling the summer squash lengthwise. The squash ribbons will resemble the wide pasta, pappardelle.
2. Combine the ricotta cheese, mint, parsley, lemon zest, lemon juice, salt, and black pepper.
3. Place mounds of the squash ribbons evenly on 4 plates then dollop the ricotta mixture on top. Drizzle with the olive oil and garnish with the mint leaves.

Nutrition:

Calories 90

Fat 6g

Carbs 5g

Protein 5g

386. Sautéed Kale with Tomato and Garlic

Preparation Time: 5 minutes

Cooking Time: 10 minutes

Servings: 4

Ingredients:

- 1 tablespoon extra-virgin olive oil
- 4 garlic cloves, sliced
- ¼ teaspoon red pepper flakes
- 2 bunches kale, stemmed and chopped or torn into pieces
- 1 (14.5-ounce) can no-salt-added diced tomatoes
- ½ teaspoon kosher salt

Directions:

1. Heat the olive oil on medium-high heat. Add the garlic, red pepper flakes, and sauté until fragrant, about 30 seconds. Add the kale and sauté, about 3 to 5 minutes, until the kale shrinks down a bit.
2. Add the tomatoes and the salt, stir together, and cook for 3 to 5 minutes, or until the liquid reduces and the kale cooks down further and becomes tender.

Nutrition:

Calories 110

Fat 5g

Carbs 15g

Protein 6g

387. Roasted Broccoli with Tahini Yogurt Sauce

Preparation Time: 15 minutes

Cooking Time: 30 minutes

Servings: 4

Ingredients:

FOR THE BROCCOLI

- 1½ to 2 pounds broccoli
- 1 lemon, sliced into ¼-inch-thick rounds
- 3 tablespoons extra-virgin olive oil
- ½ teaspoon kosher salt
- ¼ teaspoon freshly ground black pepper

FOR THE TAHINI YOGURT SAUCE

- ½ cup plain Greek yogurt

- 2 tablespoons tahini
- 1 tablespoon lemon juice
- ¼ teaspoon kosher salt
- 1 teaspoon sesame seeds, for garnish (optional)

Directions:

1. TO MAKE THE BROCCOLI
2. Preheat the oven to 425°F. Line a single baking sheet with a parchment paper or foil.
3. In a large bowl, gently toss the broccoli, lemon slices, olive oil, salt, and black pepper to combine. Lay out the broccoli in a layer on the prepared baking sheet. Roast it for about 15 minutes, stir, and roast another 15 minutes until golden brown.
4. TO MAKE THE TAHINI YOGURT SAUCE
5. Combine the yogurt, tahini, lemon juice, and salt; mix well.
6. Spread the tahini yogurt sauce on a platter or large plate and top with the broccoli and lemon slices. Garnish with the sesame seeds (if desired).

Nutrition:

Calories 245

Fat 16g

Carbs 20g

Protein 12g

388.   Green Beans with Pine Nuts and Garlic

Preparation Time: 10 minutes

Cooking Time: 20 minutes

Servings: 4-6

Ingredients:

- 1-pound green beans, trimmed
- 1 head garlic (10 to 12 cloves), smashed
- 2 tablespoons extra-virgin olive oil
- ½ teaspoon kosher salt
- ¼ teaspoon red pepper flakes
- 1 tablespoon white wine vinegar
- ¼ cup pine nuts, toasted

Directions:

1. Preheat the oven to 425°F. Line a single baking sheet with a parchment a paper or foil.
2. Combine the green beans, garlic, olive oil, salt, and red pepper flakes and mix together. Arrange it on a single layer on the baking sheet. Roast for 10 minutes, stir, and roast for another 10 minutes, or until golden brown.
3. Mix the cooked green beans with the vinegar and top with the pine nuts.

Nutrition:

Calories 165

Fat 13g

Carbs 12g

Protein 4g

389.   Roasted Harissa Carrots

Preparation Time: 10 minutes

Cooking Time: 15 minutes

Servings: 4

Ingredients:

- 1-pound carrots, peeled and sliced into 1-inch-thick rounds
- 2 tablespoons extra-virgin olive oil
- 2 tablespoons harissa
- 1 teaspoon honey
- 1 teaspoon ground cumin
- ½ teaspoon kosher salt
- ½ cup fresh parsley, chopped

Directions:

1. Preheat the oven to 450°F. Line a single baking sheet with a parchment paper or foil.
2. In a large bowl, combine the carrots, olive oil, harissa, honey, cumin, and salt. Arrange it on a single layer on the baking sheet. Roast for 15 minutes. Remove from the oven, add the parsley, and toss together.

Nutrition:

Calories 120

Fat 8g

Carbs 13g

Protein 1g

390. Cucumbers with Feta, Mint, and Sumac

Preparation Time: 15 minutes

Cooking Time: None

Servings: 4

Ingredients:

- 1 tablespoon extra-virgin olive oil
- 1 tablespoon lemon juice
- 2 teaspoons ground sumac
- ½ teaspoon kosher salt
- 2 hothouse or English cucumbers, diced
- ¼ cup crumbled feta cheese
- 1 tablespoon fresh mint, chopped
- 1 tablespoon fresh parsley, chopped
- ⅛ teaspoon red pepper flakes

Directions:

1. Add together the lemon juice, olive oil, sumac, and the salt. Add the cucumber and feta cheese and toss well.
2. Transfer it to a serving dish and then sprinkle it with the mint, parsley, and red pepper flakes.

Nutrition:

Calories 85

Fat 6g

Carbs 8g

Protein 3g

391. Cherry Tomato Bruschetta

Preparation Time: 15 minutes

Cooking Time: None

Servings: 4

Ingredients:

- 8 ounces assorted cherry tomatoes, halved

- ⅓ cup fresh herbs, chopped (such as basil, parsley, tarragon, dill)
- 1 tablespoon extra-virgin olive oil
- ¼ teaspoon kosher salt
- ⅛ teaspoon freshly ground black pepper
- ¼ cup ricotta cheese
- 4 slices whole-wheat bread, toasted

Directions:

1. Combine the tomatoes, herbs, olive oil, salt, and black pepper in a medium bowl and mix gently.
2. Spread 1 table spoon of ricotta cheese onto each slice of toast. Spoon one-quarter of the tomato mixture onto each bruschetta. If desired, garnish with more herbs.

Nutrition:

Calories 100

Fat 6g

Carbs 10g

Protein 4g

392. Roasted Red Pepper Hummus

Preparation Time: 15 minutes

Cooking Time: None

Servings: 2 cups

Ingredients:

- 1 (15-ounce) can low-sodium chickpeas, drained and rinsed
- 3 ounces jarred roasted red bell peppers, drained
- 3 tablespoons tahini
- 3 tablespoons lemon juice
- 1 garlic clove, peeled
- ¾ teaspoon kosher salt
- ¼ teaspoon freshly ground black pepper
- 3 tablespoons extra-virgin olive oil
- ¼ teaspoon cayenne pepper (optional)
- Fresh herbs, chopped, for garnish (optional)

Directions:

1. In a food processor, add the chickpeas, red bell peppers, tahini, lemon juice, garlic, salt, and black pepper. Pulse 5 to 7 times. Add the olive oil and then process until smooth. Add the cayenne pepper and garnish with chopped herbs, if desired.

Nutrition:

Calories 130

Fat 8g

Carbs 11g

Protein 4g

393. Baked Eggplant Baba Ganoush

Preparation Time: 10 minutes

Cooking Time: 1 hour

Makes about 4 cups

Ingredients:

- 2 pounds (about 2 medium to large) eggplant
- 3 tablespoons tahini
- Zest of 1 lemon
- 2 tablespoons lemon juice
- ¾ teaspoon kosher salt
- ½ teaspoon ground sumac, plus more for sprinkling (optional)
- ⅓ cup fresh parsley, chopped
- 1 tablespoon extra-virgin olive oil

Directions:

1. Preheat the oven to 350°F. Put the eggplants directly on the rack and bake for 60 minutes, or until the skin is wrinkly.
2. Add the tahini, lemon zest, lemon juice, salt, and sumac. Carefully cut open the baked eggplant and scoop the flesh into the food processor. Process until the ingredients are well blended.
3. Place in a serving dish and mix in the parsley. Drizzle it with the olive oil and then sprinkle with sumac, if desired.

Nutrition:

Calories 50

Fat 4g

Carbs 2g

Protein 1g

394. White Bean Romesco Dip

Preparation Time: 10 minutes

Cooking Time: None

Servings: 4 cups

Ingredients:

- 2 red bell peppers, or 1 (12-ounce) jar roasted sweet red peppers in water, drained
- 2 garlic cloves, peeled
- ½ cup roasted unsalted almonds
- 1 6-inch multigrain pita, torn into small pieces
- 1 teaspoon red pepper flakes
- 1 (14.5-ounce) can no-salt-added diced tomatoes
- 1 (14.5-ounce) can low-sodium cannellini beans, drained and rinsed
- 1 tablespoon fresh parsley, chopped
- 1 teaspoon sweet or smoked paprika
- 1 teaspoon kosher salt
- ¼ teaspoon black pepper
- ¼ cup extra-virgin olive oil
- 2 tablespoons red wine vinegar
- 2 teaspoons lemon juice (optional)

Directions:

1. If you are using raw peppers, roast them following the steps, then roughly chop. If using jarred roasted peppers, proceed to step 2.
2. In a food processor, add the garlic and pulse until finely minced. Sweep down the sides of the bowl and then add the almonds, pita, and red pepper flakes, and process until minced. Sweep down the sides of the bowl and then add the bell

peppers, tomatoes, beans, parsley, paprika, salt, and black pepper. Process until smooth.

3. While the food processor running, add the olive oil and vinegar, and process until smooth. Taste, and add the lemon juice to brighten, if desired.

Nutrition:

Calories 180

Fat 10g

Carbs 20g

Protein 6g

395. Roasted Cherry Tomato Caprese

Preparation Time: 15 minutes

Cooking Time: 30 minutes

Servings: 4

Ingredients:

- 2 pints (about 20 ounces) cherry tomatoes
- 6 thyme sprigs
- 6 garlic cloves, smashed
- 2 tablespoons extra-virgin olive oil
- ½ teaspoon kosher salt
- 8 ounces fresh, unsalted mozzarella, cut into bite-size slices
- ¼ cup basil, chopped or cut into ribbons
- Loaf of crusty whole-wheat bread for serving

Directions:

1. Preheat the oven to 350°F. Line a single baking sheet with a parchment paper or foil.
2. Put the tomatoes, thyme, garlic, olive oil, and salt into a large bowl and mix together. Put it on the prepared baking sheet in a single layer. Roast for 30 minutes, or until the tomatoes are bursting and juicy.

3. Place the mozzarella on a platter or in a bowl. Pour all the tomato mixture, including the juices, over the mozzarella. Garnish with the basil.
4. Serve with crusty bread.

Nutrition:

Calories 250

Fat 17g

Carbs 9g

Protein 17g

396. Italian Crepe with Herbs and Onion

Preparation Time: 15 minutes + 30 minutes to rest

Cooking Time: 20 minutes per crepe

Servings: 6

Ingredients:

- 2 cups cold water
- 1 cup chickpea flour
- ½ teaspoon kosher salt
- ¼ teaspoon freshly ground black pepper
- 3½ tablespoons extra-virgin olive oil, divided
- ½ onion, julienned
- ½ cup fresh herbs, chopped (thyme, sage, and rosemary are all nice on their own or as a mix)

Directions:

1. In a large bowl, whisk together the water, flour, salt, and black pepper. Add 2 tablespoons of the olive oil and whisk. Allow the batter sit at room temperature for at least 30 minutes.
2. Preheat the oven to 450°F. Place a 12-inch cast-iron pan or oven-safe skillet in the oven to warm as the oven comes to temperature.
3. Put away the hot pan from the oven carefully, add ½ tablespoon of the olive oil and one-third of the onion, stir, and place the pan back in the oven. Cook

while stirring it occasionally, until the onions are golden brown, 5 to 8 minutes.

4. Remove the pan from the oven and pour in one-third of the batter (about 1 cup), sprinkle with one-third of the herbs, and put it back in the oven. Bake for 10 minutes, or until firm and the edges are set.
5. Increase the oven setting to broil and cook 3 to 5 minutes, or until golden brown. Slide the crepe onto the cutting board and repeat twice more. Halve the crepes and cut into wedges. Serve warm or at room temperature.

Nutrition:

Calories 135

Fat 9g

Carbs 11g

Protein 4g

397. Light & Creamy Garlic Hummus

Preparation Time: 10 minutes

Cooking Time: 40 minutes

Servings: 12

Ingredients:

- 1 1/2 cups dry chickpeas, rinsed
- 2 1/2 tbsp fresh lemon juice
- 1 tbsp garlic, minced
- 1/2 cup tahini
- 6 cups of water
- Pepper
- Salt

Directions:

1. Add water and chickpeas into the instant pot.
2. Seal pot with a lid and select manual and set timer for 40 minutes.
3. Once done, allow to release pressure naturally. Remove lid.
4. Drain chickpeas well and reserved 1/2 cup chickpeas liquid.

5. Transfer chickpeas, reserved liquid, lemon juice, garlic, tahini, pepper, and salt into the food processor and process until smooth.
6. Serve and enjoy.

Nutrition:

Calories: 152

Fat: 6.9g

Carbs: 17.6g

Protein: 6.6g

398. Perfect Queso

Preparation Time: 10 minutes

Cooking Time: 15 minutes

Servings: 16

Ingredients:

- 1 lb. ground beef
- 32 oz Velveeta cheese, cut into cubes
- 10 oz can tomato, diced
- 1 1/2 tbsp taco seasoning
- 1 tsp chili powder
- 1 onion, diced
- Pepper
- Salt

Directions:

1. Set instant pot on sauté mode.
2. Add meat, onion, taco seasoning, chili powder, pepper, and salt into the pot and cook until meat is no longer pink.
3. Add tomatoes and stir well. Top with cheese and do not stir.
4. Seal pot with a lid and then cook it on high for 4 minutes.
5. Once done, release pressure using quick release. Remove lid.
6. Stir everything well and serve.

Nutrition:

Calories: 257

Fat: 15.9g

Carbs: 10.2g

Protein: 21g

399. Creamy Potato Spread

Preparation Time: 10 minutes

Cooking Time: 15 minutes

Servings: 6

Ingredients:

- 1 lb. sweet potatoes, peeled and chopped
- 3/4 tbsp fresh chives, chopped
- 1/2 tsp paprika
- 1 tbsp garlic, minced
- 1 cup tomato puree
- Pepper
- Salt

Directions:

1. Add all ingredients except chives into the inner pot of instant pot and stir well.
2. Seal pot with lid and cook on high for 15 minutes.
3. Once done, allow to release pressure naturally for 10 minutes then release remaining using quick release. Remove lid.
4. Transfer instant pot sweet potato mixture into the food processor and process until smooth.
5. Garnish with chives and serve.

Nutrition:

Calories: 108

Fat: 0.3g

Carbs: 25.4g

Protein: 2g

400. Cucumber Tomato Okra Salsa

Preparation Time: 10 minutes

Cooking Time: 15 minutes

Servings: 4

Ingredients:

- 1 lb. tomatoes, chopped
- 1/4 tsp red pepper flakes
- 1/4 cup fresh lemon juice
- 1 cucumber, chopped
- 1 tbsp fresh oregano, chopped
- 1 tbsp fresh basil, chopped
- 1 tbsp olive oil
- 1 onion, chopped
- 1 tbsp garlic, chopped
- 1 1/2 cups okra, chopped
- Pepper
- Salt

Directions:

1. Add oil into the inner pot of instant pot and set the pot on sauté mode.
2. Add onion, garlic, pepper, and salt and sauté for 3 minutes.
3. Add remaining ingredients except for cucumber and stir well.
4. Seal pot with lid and cook on high for 12 minutes.
5. Once done, allow to release pressure naturally for 10 minutes then release remaining using quick release. Remove lid.
6. Once the salsa mixture is cool then add cucumber and mix well.
7. Serve and enjoy.

Nutrition:

Calories: 99

Fat: 4.2g

Carbs: 14.3g

Protein: 2.9g

401. Parmesan Potatoes

Preparation Time: 10 minutes

Cooking Time: 6 minutes

Servings: 4

Ingredients:

- 2 lb. potatoes, rinsed and cut into chunks
- 2 tbsp parmesan cheese, grated

- 2 tbsp olive oil
- 1/2 tsp parsley
- 1/2 tsp Italian seasoning
- 1 tsp garlic, minced
- 1 cup vegetable broth
- 1/2 tsp salt

Directions:

1. Add all ingredients except cheese into the instant pot and stir well.
2. Seal pot with lid and cook on high for 6 minutes.
3. Once done, release pressure using quick release. Remove lid.
4. Add parmesan cheese and stir until cheese is melted.
5. Serve and enjoy.

Nutrition:

Calories: 237

Fat: 8.3g

Carbs: 36.3g

Protein: 5.9g

402.   Creamy Artichoke Dip

Preparation Time: 10 minutes

Cooking Time: 5 minutes

Servings: 8

Ingredients:

- 28 oz can artichoke hearts, drain and quartered
- 1 1/2 cups parmesan cheese, shredded
- 1 cup sour cream
- 1 cup mayonnaise
  - oz can green chilies
- 1 cup of water
- Pepper
- Salt

Directions:

1. Add artichokes, water, and green chilis into the instant pot.

2. Seal pot with the lid and select manual and set timer for 1 minute.
3. Once done, release pressure using quick release. Remove lid. Drain excess water.
4. Set instant pot on sauté mode. Add remaining ingredients and stir well and cook until cheese is melted.
5. Serve and enjoy.

Nutrition:

Calories: 262

Fat: 7.6g

Carbs: 14.4g

Protein: 8.4g

403.   Homemade Salsa

Preparation Time: 10 minutes

Cooking Time: 5 minutes

Servings: 8

Ingredients:

- 12 oz grape tomatoes, halved
- 1/4 cup fresh cilantro, chopped
- 1 fresh lime juice
- 28 oz tomatoes, crushed
- 1 tbsp garlic, minced
- 1 green bell pepper, chopped
- 1 red bell pepper, chopped
- 2 onions, chopped
- 6 whole tomatoes
- Salt

Directions:

1. Add whole tomatoes into the instant pot and gently smash the tomatoes.
2. Add remaining ingredients except cilantro, lime juice, and salt and stir well.
3. Seal pot with lid and cook on high for 5 minutes.
4. Once done, allow to release pressure naturally for 10 minutes then release remaining using quick release. Remove lid.
5. Add cilantro, lime juice, and salt and stir well.

6. Serve and enjoy.

Nutrition:

Calories: 146

Fat: 1.2g

Carbs: 33.2g

Protein: 6.9g

404. Delicious Eggplant Caponata

Preparation Time: 10 minutes

Cooking Time: 5 minutes

Servings: 8

Ingredients:

- 1 eggplant, cut into 1/2-inch chunks
- 1 lb. tomatoes, diced
- 1/2 cup tomato puree
- 1/4 cup dates, chopped
- 2 tbsp vinegar
- 1/2 cup fresh parsley, chopped
- 2 celery stalks, chopped
- 1 small onion, chopped
- 2 zucchini, cut into 1/2-inch chunks
- Pepper
- Salt

Directions:

1. Add all ingredients into the inner pot of instant pot and stir well.
2. Seal pot with lid and cook on high for 5 minutes.
3. Once done, release pressure using quick release. Remove lid.
4. Stir well and serve.

Nutrition:

Calories: 60

Fat: 0.4g

Carbs: 14g

Protein: 2.3g

405. Flavorful Roasted Baby Potatoes

Preparation Time: 10 minutes

Cooking Time: 10 minutes

Servings: 4

Ingredients:

- 2 lbs. baby potatoes, clean and cut in half
- 1/2 cup vegetable stock
- 1 tsp paprika
- 3/4 tsp garlic powder
- 1 tsp onion powder
- 2 tsp Italian seasoning
- 1 tbsp olive oil
- Pepper
- Salt

Directions:

1. Add oil into the inner pot of instant pot and set the pot on sauté mode.
2. Add potatoes and sauté for 5 minutes. Add remaining ingredients and stir well.
3. Seal pot with lid and cook on high for 5 minutes.
4. Once done, release pressure using quick release. Remove lid.
5. Stir well and serve.

Nutrition:

Calories: 175

Fat: 4.5g

Carbs: 29.8g

Protein: 6.1g

406. Perfect Italian Potatoes

Preparation Time: 10 minutes

Cooking Time: 7 minutes

Servings: 6

Ingredients:

- 2 lbs. baby potatoes, clean and cut in half
- 3/4 cup vegetable broth

- 6 oz Italian dry dressing mix

Directions:

1. Add all ingredients into the inner pot of instant pot and stir well.
2. Seal pot with lid and cook on high for 7 minutes.
3. Once done, allow to release pressure naturally for 3 minutes then release remaining using quick release. Remove lid.
4. Stir well and serve.

Nutrition:

Calories: 149

Fat: 0.3g

Carbs: 41.6g

Protein: 4.5g

407. Garlic Pinto Bean Dip

Preparation Time: 10 minutes

Cooking Time: 43 minutes

Servings: 6

Ingredients:

- 1 cup dry pinto beans, rinsed
- 1/2 tsp cumin
- 1/2 cup salsa
- 2 garlic cloves
- 2 chipotle peppers in adobo sauce
- 5 cups vegetable stock
- Pepper
- Salt

Directions:

1. Add beans, stock, garlic, and chipotle peppers into the instant pot.
2. Seal the pot with a lid and cook on high for 43 minutes.
3. Once done, release pressure using quick release. Remove lid.
4. Drain beans well and reserve 1/2 cup of stock.

5. Transfer beans, reserve stock, and remaining ingredients into the food processor and process until smooth.
6. Serve and enjoy.

Nutrition:

Calories: 129

Fat: 0.9g

Carbs: 23g

Protein: 8g

408. Creamy Eggplant Dip

Preparation Time: 10 minutes

Cooking Time: 20 minutes

Servings: 4

Ingredients:

- 1 eggplant
- 1/2 tsp paprika
- 1 tbsp olive oil
- 1 tbsp fresh lime juice
- 2 tbsp tahini
- 1 garlic clove
- 1 cup of water
- Pepper
- Salt

Directions:

1. Add water and eggplant into the instant pot.
2. Seal pot with the lid and select manual and set timer for 20 minutes.
3. Once done, release pressure using quick release. Remove lid.
4. Drain eggplant and let it cool.
5. Once the eggplant is cool then remove eggplant skin and transfer eggplant flesh into the food processor.
6. Add remaining ingredients into the food processor and process until smooth.
7. Serve and enjoy.

Nutrition:

Calories: 108

Fat: 7.8g

Carbs: 9.7g

Protein: 2.5g

409. Jalapeno Chickpea Hummus

Preparation Time: 10 minutes

Cooking Time: 25 minutes

Servings: 4

Ingredients:

- 1 cup dry chickpeas, soaked overnight and drained
- 1 tsp ground cumin
- 1/4 cup jalapenos, diced
- 1/2 cup fresh cilantro
- 1 tbsp tahini
- 1/2 cup olive oil
- Pepper
- Salt

Directions:

1. Add chickpeas into the instant pot and cover with vegetable stock.
2. Seal the pot a with lid and then cook on high for 25 minutes.
3. Once done, allow to release pressure naturally. Remove lid.
4. Drain chickpeas well and transfer into the food processor along with remaining ingredients and process until smooth.
5. Serve and enjoy.

Nutrition:

Calories: 425

Fat: 30.4g

Carbs: 31.8g

Protein: 10.5g

410. Tasty Black Bean Dip

Preparation Time: 10 minutes

Cooking Time: 18 minutes

Servings: 6

Ingredients:

- 2 cups dry black beans, soaked overnight and drained
- 1 1/2 cups cheese, shredded
- 1 tsp dried oregano
- 1 1/2 tsp chili powder
- 2 cups tomatoes, chopped
- 2 tbsp olive oil
- 1 1/2 tbsp garlic, minced
- 1 medium onion, sliced
- 4 cups vegetable stock
- Pepper
- Salt

Directions:

1. Add all ingredients except cheese into the instant pot.
2. Seal pot with lid and cook on high for 18 minutes.
3. Once done, allow to release pressure naturally. Remove lid. Drain excess water.
4. Add cheese and stir until cheese is melted.
5. Blend bean mixture using an immersion blender until smooth.
6. Serve and enjoy.

Nutrition:

Calories: 402

Fat: 15.3g

Carbs: 46.6g

Protein: 22.2g

411. Healthy Kidney Bean Dip

Preparation Time: 10 minutes

Cooking Time: 10 minutes

Servings: 6

Ingredients:

- 1 cup dry white kidney beans, soaked overnight and drained
- 1 tbsp fresh lemon juice

- 2 tbsp water
- 1/2 cup coconut yogurt
- 1 roasted garlic clove
- 1 tbsp olive oil
- 1/4 tsp cayenne
- 1 tsp dried parsley
- Pepper
- Salt

Directions:

1. Add soaked beans and 1 3/4 cups of water into the instant pot.
2. Seal the pot with a lid and then cook on high for 10 minutes.
3. Once done, allow to release pressure naturally. Remove lid.
4. Drain beans well and transfer them into the food processor.
5. Add left ingredients into the food processor and then process until smooth.
6. Serve and enjoy.

Nutrition:

Calories: 136

Fat: 3.2g

Carbs: 20g

Protein: 7.7g

412.   Creamy Pepper Spread

Preparation Time: 10 minutes

Cooking Time: 15 minutes

Servings: 4

Ingredients:

- 1 lb. red bell peppers, chopped and remove seeds
- 1 1/2 tbsp fresh basil
- 1 tbsp olive oil
- 1 tbsp fresh lime juice
- 1 tsp garlic, minced
- Pepper
- Salt

Directions:

1. Add all ingredients into the inner pot of instant pot and stir well.
2. Seal pot with lid and cook on high for 15 minutes.
3. Once done, allow to release pressure naturally for 10 minutes then release remaining using quick release. Remove lid.
4. Transfer bell pepper mixture into the food processor and process until smooth.
5. Serve and enjoy.

Nutrition:

Calories: 41

Fat: 3.6g

Carbs: 3.5g

Protein: 0.4g

413.   Baba Ganoush

Preparation Time: 10 minutes

Cooking Time: 15 minutes

Servings: 6

Ingredients:

- 1 eggplant, peeled and sliced
- ¼ cup tahini
- ½ teaspoon sea salt
- Juice of 1 lemon
- ¼ teaspoon ground cumin
- ⅛ teaspoon freshly ground black pepper
- 2 tablespoons extra-virgin olive oil
- 2 tablespoons sunflower seeds (optional)
- 2 tablespoons fresh Italian parsley leaves (optional)

Directions:

1. Preheat the oven to 350°F.
2. On a baking sheet, spread the eggplant slices in an even layer. Bake for about 15 minutes until soft. Cool slightly and roughly chop the eggplant.
3. In a blender, blend the eggplant with the tahini, sea salt, lemon juice, cumin, and pepper for about 30 seconds. Transfer to a serving dish.

4. Drizzle with the olive oil and sprinkle with the sunflower seeds and parsley (if using) before serving.

Nutrition:

Calories: 121

Fat: 10g

Carbs: 7g

Protein: 3g

Measurement Conversion Chart

DRY WEIGHTS

1/2 oz	1 tbsp	-	15 g
1 oz	2 tbsp	1/8 c	28 g
2 oz	4 tbsp	1/4 c	57 g
3 oz	6 tbsp	1/3 c	85 g
4 oz	8 tbsp	1/2 c	115 g
8 oz	16 tbsp	1 cup	227 g
12 oz	24 tbsp	1½ c	340 g
16 oz	32 tbsp	2 c	455 g

1 OZ = 28 GRAMS
1 LBS = 454 G
1 CUP = 227 G

1 TSP = 5 ML
1 TBSP = 15 ML
1 OZ = 30 ML
1 CUP = 237 ML
1 PINT = 473 ML (2 CUPS)
1 GALLON = 16 CUPS

LIQUID VOLUMES

1 oz	2 tbsp	1/8 c	30 ml
2 oz	4 tbsp	1/4 c	60 ml
2⅔ oz	6 tbsp	1/3 c	80 ml
4 oz	8 tbsp	1/2 c	120 ml
8 oz	16 tbsp	2/3 c	160 ml
12 oz	24 tbsp	3/4 c	177 ml
16 oz	32 tbsp	1 cup	237 ml
32 oz	64 tbsp	1½ c	470 ml
		2 c	950 ml

ABBREVIATIONS

tbsp = Tablespoon
tsp = Teaspoon
fl.oz = Fluid Ounce
c = cup
ml = Milliliter
lb = pound
F = Fahrenheit
C = Celsius
ml = Milliliter
g = grams
kg = kilogram
l = liter

BAKING PAN

9-inch (by 3") standard round pan = 12 cups
9-inch (by 2.5") springform pan = 10 cups
10-inch (by 4") tube pan = 16 cups
9-inch (by 3") bundt pan = 12 cups
9-inch (by 2") square pan = 10 cups
9 x 5 inch loaf pan = 8 cups

OVEN TEMP.

130 c = 250 F
165 c = 325 F
177 c = 350 F
190 c = 375 F
200 c = 400 F
220 c = 425 F

Conclusion

In the past, the Mediterranean Diet and its benefits have been extensively studied with focus on cardiovascular disease and obesity. The evidence for a Mediterranean diet is clear, but whether or not it provides an overall health advantage or simply reduces risk factors remains debatable. A recent meta-analysis published in the Annals of Internal Medicine found that following the Mediterranean Diet reduces heart attack risk by 22%. It also found that diets rich in vegetables, fruit, nuts and non-processed foods reduced all cause mortality by 12% compared to low-fat diets like Atkins. This study built on previous large scale meta analyses which demonstrated a 20% reduction in heart disease risk after following this type of diet over 10 years. While the Mediterranean Diet is not associated with increased cancer risk, smaller studies have shown that following a Mediterranean diet is associated with a lower risk of cancer up to 30%. This higher cancer risk reduction is explained by the fact that following the Mediterranean Diet often means more red meat, saturated fat and sodium are consumed. These higher intakes have been associated with an increased breast cancer risk. Although this recent meta-analysis re-affirmed previous research on the benefits of the Mediterranean Diet, it did not answer some key questions. The study did not look at vegan diets and whether or not they provided similar benefits as a high vegetable, fruit and olive oil intake. Another important question is how much of a health benefit to the Mediterranean Diet actually depends on the quality of food consumed. Often supplements are added to plant based diets, but these can hinder the overall body's ability to absorb vitamins and minerals for optimal health. While this study found that following a Mediterranean Diet help reduce all-cause mortality by 12%, it did not account for these lifestyle differences.

The main difference between the Mediterranean Diet and other popular diets is that it avoids foods high in saturated fat, salt and cholesterol. It also focuses on eating a greater amount of vegetables, fruit, nuts and unprocessed carbohydrates from whole grains. The diet discourages meat consumption and has a high omega-3 fatty acid intake, which is thought to reduce the risk of heart disease. The Mediterranean Diet also emphasizes eating meals with family and friends. The traditional Mediterranean Diet is rich in vegetables, fruits, legumes, whole grains, fish and healthy fats such as virgin olive oil. A traditional diet also contains moderate amounts of red wine. However, wine has been removed from the modern interpretation of this diet due to its high sugar content.

The Mediterranean Diet is low in red meat and saturated fat consumption when compared to other diets like low-carb, high protein diets or the Atkins eating plan. For this reason, the Mediterranean Diet has been associated with a reduced all-cause mortality. There are also no significant differences between the Mediterranean Diet and other high protein, low cholesterol, low saturated fat diets in terms of cardiovascular disease risk. While there is no evidence suggesting that following a Mediterranean Diet will lead to a reduction in cancer or overall mortality, there is some evidence explaining why. The traditional interpretation of this diet limits red meat and saturated fat intake, which are known to increase the risk of heart disease in those who do not have heart disease. This diet also limits dietary cholesterol intake and encourages consumption of fruits and vegetables, which have been associated with a reduced risk of cancer.

Printed in Great Britain
by Amazon